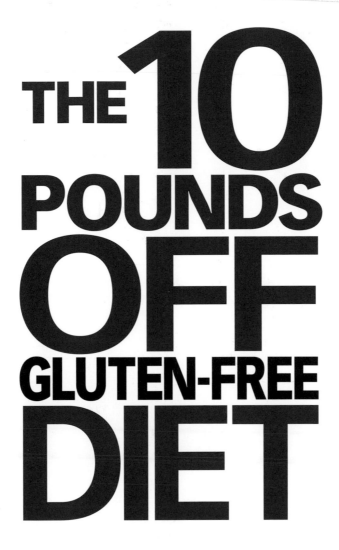

THE 10 POUNDS OFF GLUTEN-FREE DIET

From the experts at CookingLight

THE 10 POUNDS OFF GLUTEN-FREE DIET

The Easy Way to Drop Inches in Just 28 Days

Oxmoor House

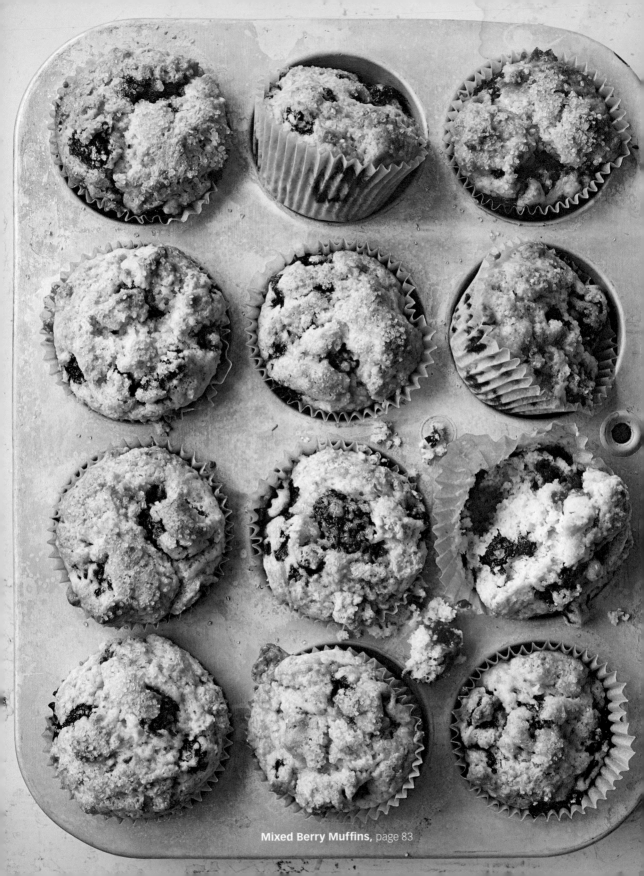

Mixed Berry Muffins, page 83

CONTENTS

INTRODUCTION 6

PART 1 **GLUTEN-FREE POWER**

GLUTEN FREE AND YOUR HEALTH 10

WHY GOING GLUTEN FREE IS GOOD FOR YOU 20

THE NUTS AND BOLTS OF GOING GLUTEN FREE 28

PUTTING YOUR GLUTEN-FREE DIET INTO ACTION 42

TAKE THE GLUTEN-FREE DIET CHALLENGE 50

PART 2 **100 GLUTEN-FREE RECIPES**

GLUTEN-FREE SHOPPING LIST 62

BREAKFAST 66

LUNCH 86

DINNER 106

SNACKS & SIDES 144

DESSERTS 164

PART 3 **LIVING THE GLUTEN-FREE LIFESTYLE**

EXERCISING FOR GLUTEN-FREE HEALTH 188

MAINTAIN YOUR GAINS THE GLUTEN-FREE WAY 202

MIND-BODY JOURNAL 210

NUTRITIONAL INFORMATION AND METRIC EQUIVALENTS 220

REFERENCES 221

INDEX 222

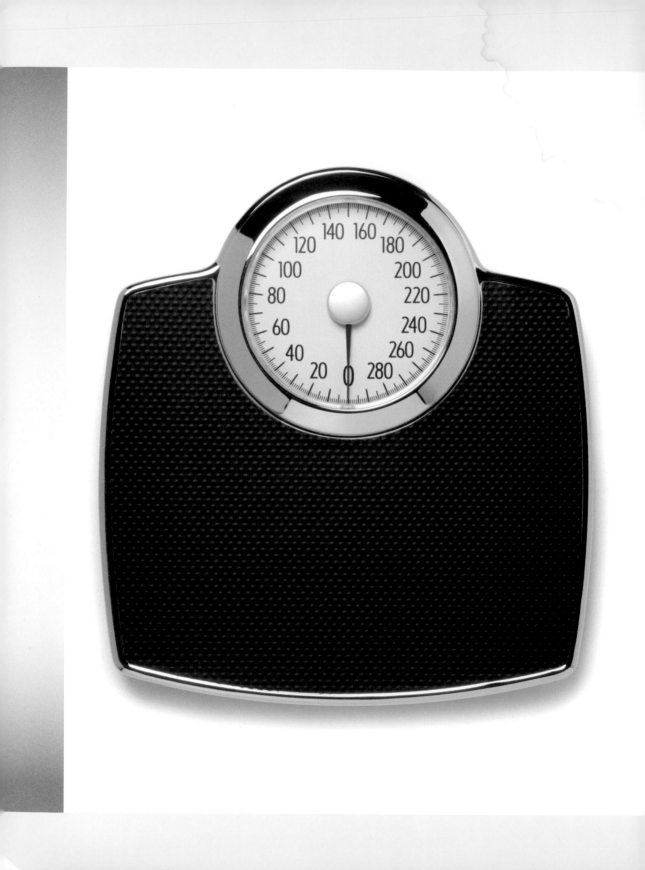

WHO DOESN'T WANT TO SEE THE SCALE 10 POUNDS LIGHTER?

This book will show you how to do just that while adhering to a gluten-free eating plan. In the following pages, you'll find a comprehensive introduction to the diet (complete with cutting-edge research) as well as 100 recipes from the healthy cooking experts at *Cooking Light,* four weeks of meal plans, and a do-anywhere fitness plan to help you tone up and slim down—safely, easily, and deliciously.

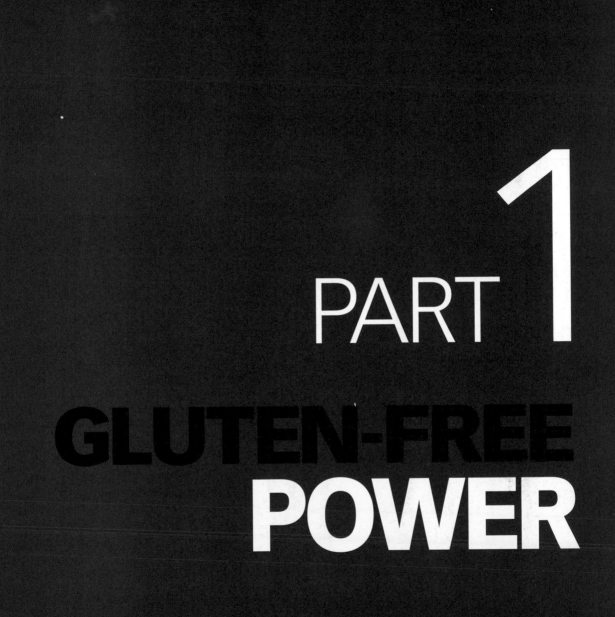

PART 1

GLUTEN-FREE POWER

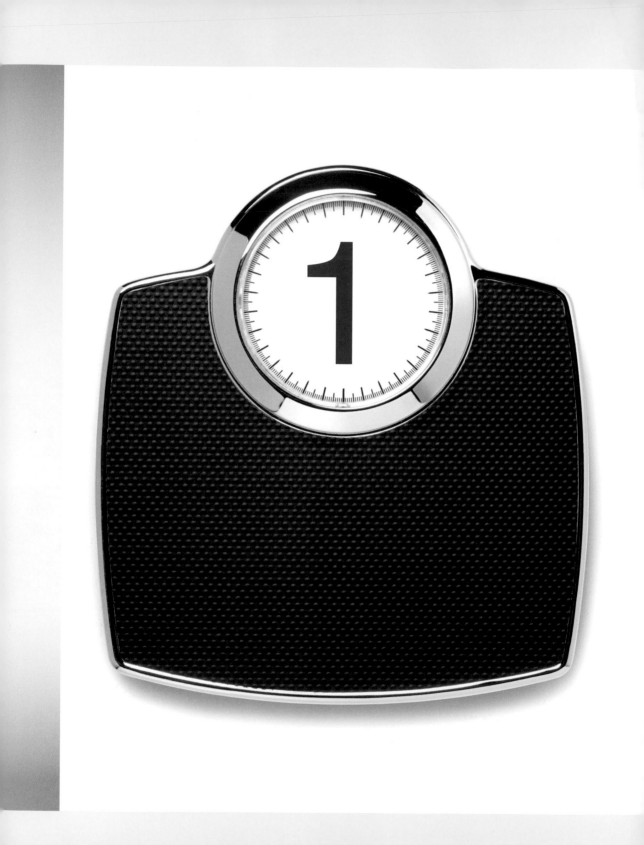

GLUTEN HAS BEEN A BUZZ-WORD FOR THE LAST FEW YEARS. You probably know people who have gone gluten free and wondered what it might do for you. As a diet concept, going gluten free has been increasing by leaps and bounds. You can find gluten-free foods at most supermarkets, delis, and restaurants. There is even gluten-free beer, which is quite a trick when you consider the importance of gluten-containing barley to the beer-making process.

Helpful definitions
• *Celiac disease* is a genetic disorder in which gluten damages the lining of the small intestine, leading to a number of physical and neurological symptoms that vary from person to person. Gluten must be avoided for life.
• *Gluten sensitivity* (GS) and *gluten intolerance* (GI) are often used interchangeably. Individuals have trouble digesting gluten and don't feel well after eating it. While these conditions share some of the same symptoms of celiac disease, GI and GS patients have not shown damage to their small intestine.
• A *wheat allergy* causes an allergic reaction to wheat, but people with this allergy may be able to tolerate other grains, such as oats, rye, and barley, since the allergy is not in response to gluten.

Gluten is a combination of proteins found in wheat, barley, rye, and triticale (a wheat/rye hybrid). In bread making, gluten develops as the dough is kneaded, making it springier. For some people, the protein can cause severe difficulties with their digestive tract (more about that later). Others believe that they might have a sensitivity to gluten that could be causing them to gain weight or suffer achy joints and headaches, among other health problems.

Individuals with celiac disease, which is an immune response to gluten, have difficulty absorbing nutrients from certain foods and may end up *losing* weight, not gaining it. Those with gluten sensitivity, whose symptoms include diarrhea or abdominal pain, may also lose weight prior to restricting gluten from their diet, but others with gluten-related issues may still struggle with their weight. If you suspect you have celiac disease or a wheat allergy, you should speak to a medical professional to get the appropriate testing done before going on a gluten-free diet. (There is no diagnostic test to confirm gluten sensitivity or gluten intolerance.) It's more difficult to diagnose these issues if you give up gluten before being tested. If you test negative, you could eliminate gluten from your diet to see if your symptoms improve, which would imply a gluten sensitivity.

The Perfect Way to Lose 10 Pounds

When you set out to shed just a few pounds, the last thing you want to do is adopt a complex eating system. A huge advantage of going gluten free is that you don't have to weigh food, do elaborate planning for meals, or count calories or points. That may seem liberating—or possibly a little frightening, if you're accustomed to diets with rigid calorie- or points-counting rules.

By eliminating gluten, you won't have to count calories because you'll naturally avoid many of the foods that lead to weight gain. This diet encourages you to eat whole foods and avoid highly processed foods—including the gluten-free options—that are often high in calories, refined carbohydrates, fat, and added sugar. Eating the foods you're meant to consume will help you naturally feel full before you're at risk of overeating. Plus, you'll stay satisfied for much longer than when you eat the cheap, nutritionally unfulfilling foods so common in our modern diet. Although dieting experts set the pace of safe weight loss at 2 pounds per week, once you start your gluten-free diet, you may be surprised that you lose more than that in the first several weeks.

The Right Diet for Shedding Pounds

Look, you probably know that if you eat fewer calories than you burn through exercise and daily activity, you will lose weight. But one thing researchers have learned in the last decade is that there's nothing simple about how the calories you eat influence appetite. The biggest surprise was that low-fiber carbohydrates—think of white-flour bread and crackers, and low-fat, high-sugar treats—could actually *increase* hunger. These simple, easily digested carbohydrates break down more rapidly and cause a bigger increase in your blood sugar than carbohydrates that contain more fiber and take longer to digest. The sudden surge of glucose provokes a rise in insulin, the hormone your body relies on to process sugar. All that glucose either gets burned up for energy or shuttled off to places like your thighs and belly to be converted to long-term storage—in other words, fat.

The rapid peak and then plunge in blood sugar is a source of weight-gain troubles. As levels fall, your gut signals to your brain that energy supplies are running low, and just like that, you're hungry again or have less energy. The calories you consumed are responsible for making you want to eat more, and suddenly the calories in vs. calories out equation doesn't add up the way we always thought it did.

The solution is to add more lean protein (fish, lean cuts of meat, and nuts), high-fiber carbohydrates (brown rice, amaranth, millet, and certified gluten-free oats), and healthy fats to your diet. All these foods take longer to digest, resulting in a more gradual rise of blood sugar. You'll feel full longer and give yourself a chance to tip the scale in your favor.

Beginning a new plan will fill you with energy so you may be more active. Within a week or two you'll find that your face and shape are noticeably different when you gaze in the mirror!

Lose Belly Fat Faster

Incorporating more lean protein into your gluten-free diet has some other benefits. Carrying extra pounds around the midsection may be the most troubling aspect of being overweight. Research has found that too much fat in your belly is harder on organs, arteries, and the heart than fat you carry elsewhere, such as on your hips or thighs. According to new research, diets high in protein might help you target your spare tire.

At McMaster University in Ontario, researchers recruited 90 overweight and obese women and put them on a regular exercise schedule of walking and strength training. They also assigned them to one of three diets, featuring high, medium, and low amounts of protein. The researchers measured the volunteers' fat and muscle both at the beginning of the study and four months later, at the end. While all the women lost the same amount of weight on average, the big difference was in their levels of fat

TIP

Embrace the basics. If you don't have to eat gluten free for medical reasons, you may not want to eat this way for the rest of your life. But as you make the healthy changes required by this diet (fewer processed foods, less sugar, more home cooking), embrace them as permanent changes that will keep you slim.

"When you feel better, there is a domino effect. I deal with stress better, sleep well, and no longer worry about what I'm going to eat."

Success Story:
Carmen

Carmen searched for an answer to ongoing GI problems, trying multiple physicians who repeatedly told her, "It's all in your head." Finally, one physician listened to Carmen and tested her for gluten-related conditions. He recommended she follow a gluten-free eating plan. It worked so well that she lost 13 pounds and found relief from GI flare-ups. Her orthopedic physician was thrilled with the weight loss as well, due to Carmen's hip dysplasia, which is managed more effectively at a healthy weight. The weight loss also helped Carmen achieve the highest level of fitness in her employer's wellness program and earned her a substantial financial reward.

"I feel better and don't have to worry about GI problems like I did in the past. When you feel better, there is a domino effect. I deal with stress better, sleep well, and no longer worry about what I'm going to eat. It's really freed me to live without fear of what I eat."

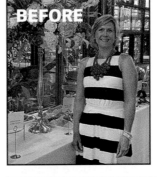

BEFORE

AFTER

Age: **42**

Height: **5'2"**

Weight before:
143

Weight after:
130

Pounds lost:
13

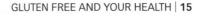

and muscle: 100 percent of the weight loss in the high-protein group was fat, especially around the midsection.

What's more, they added about a pound and half of muscle, while the low-protein group actually lost 1.5 pounds of muscle. "The preservation or even gain of muscle is very important for maintaining metabolic rate and preventing weight regain, which can be a major problem for many seeking to lose weight," says Andrea Josse, lead author of the study and a graduate student in the Department of Kinesiology at McMaster University.

How much protein did the women consume? The amounts weren't too daunting: They got about 30 percent of their calories from protein—about what you'd get on a gluten-free plan; most Americans typically get in the neighborhood of 15 to 20 percent.

TIP

Decide the best way for *you* to make a change. Some people like to remove all the off-limits food at once. Others thrive when they eliminate one food group at a time— start by getting rid of wheat, for example, then, a week or two later, processed sugars. Think about which approach sounds more appealing to you.

A study from Denmark is just the latest to underscore the importance of cutting back on carbohydrates in favor of lean, healthy protein. Nutrition researchers at the University of Copenhagen put 744 obese adults on several different diets that ranged from a traditional low-protein (13 percent of total calories) plan to one that got about 25 percent of its calories from protein. Each diet received a fairly liberal 25 to 30 percent of calories from fat.

After eight weeks, each group had lost an average of 24 pounds, although nearly 40 percent of the high-carb group dropped out, compared to just 25 percent of the high-protein group. But the true advantage to increasing protein became apparent six months later when the researchers followed up with the dieters. Those who had followed the high-carb plan had regained an average of roughly 4 pounds, while the high-protein group averaged less than 2 pounds of weight regain.

In addition to eating more healthy protein like turkey and fish, the successful dieters added quality, high-fiber carbohydrates such as brown rice, say the researchers. The advantage to high-fiber carbs is that they slow down digestion, allowing you to feel full longer. Protein also takes longer to digest—a diet composed of these foods will keep your gut busy, reducing hunger between meals.

The Benefits of a Gluten-Free Diet

Health is one of the biggest concerns—and reasons—dieters debate when adopting this plan. In fact, some researchers and diet experts still debate whether an approach that encourages protein and eliminates many carbohydrate-rich foods can really be safe. But rest assured that you can cut back on gluten for weeks or months and not worry about your health.

Obviously, a gluten-free diet offers great health benefits to those individuals diagnosed with celiac disease, gluten sensitivity, and wheat allergies; it's also sometimes recommended for children with autism. Celiac disease is a digestive disorder in which gluten damages the lining of the small intestine and reduces its ability to absorb vital nutrients. This condition is an autoimmune one rather than a food allergy, as gluten-containing food actually causes damage to the lining of the small intestine. This damage increases the risk of malnutrition because the small intestine can't effectively absorb nutrients. Common symptoms include diarrhea, constipation, gas, bloating, weight loss, nausea, vitamin deficiencies, and severe abdominal pain, but gluten can also cause further damage and additional symptoms in other areas of the body. The range and severity of symptoms varies greatly among individuals, and the level of gluten in certain foods affects each person differently. The only treatment is a lifelong gluten-free diet.

Persons with gluten sensitivity can exhibit a wide range of reactions, from digestive issues to headaches, balance problems, and many other

TIP

When you're eliminating gluten, pick up the slack with more produce. A smart thing to do when you start this plan is to make sure your house is stocked with plenty of healthy produce. Keep in-season fruit in bowls on your counters and dining table and in your fridge.

TIP

Recruit a partner.
Getting your spouse,
friend, or family
member to join you
will help you get off
to a good start. The
two of you can share
ideas and recipes,
and keep each other
on track through the
tough times. One
thing is for certain:
Taking efforts to
eliminate gluten
from your diet
will help you shed
pounds. Essentially,
you'll be eliminating
a lot of the cheap
carbohydrates that
are directly related
to weight gain. You'll
also increase your
protein intake, and
there are a lot of
good studies that
suggest that eating
high-quality, lean
protein can help you
slim down.

difficulties. And these symptoms may range from mild to severe. The only treatment for gluten sensitivity is avoidance of gluten. Individuals with allergies must avoid wheat proteins, which include gluten. Symptoms can include hives, nasal congestion, nausea, and anaphylaxis. The only treatment is avoidance of wheat products. Some physicians prescribe a diet free of gluten and casein (a milk protein) to improve behavior in children with autism. Not all autistic children respond to a gluten-free/casein-free diet (known as a GFCF diet), and it is typically used as a part of the overall treatment.

Lactose Intolerance

Some people who cannot eat gluten also experience lactose intolerance—gluten-induced damage to the intestines can decrease the ability to digest lactose. For the recipes in this book containing dairy products, you can make ingredient substitutions using dairy-free plain yogurts and cheeses, dairy-free buttery spreads in place of butter, and dairy-free beverages such as plain rice, soy, almond, coconut, or hemp milk in place of cow's milk. Please note that these products often have different textures and flavors compared to their dairy-containing counterparts, so you may need to experiment with the recipes to get the results you like.

Other Health Benefits

Weight loss alone can help reduce your risk of many chronic diseases, such as heart disease, diabetes, and several forms of cancer. By eating more healthy lean protein, gluten-free whole grains, and healthy fats, you'll go even further toward protecting yourself.

Healthy fats and proteins have surged to the forefront of good nutrition. We've come a long way from just 10 years ago, when government health experts and most major health organizations insisted that getting more than 30 percent of your calories from fat would blow you up like a balloon. Studies at Harvard revealed that people following low-fat diets lost less weight and were more likely to abandon their diets compared to people who followed regimens based on the Mediterranean diet, which contained as much as 40 percent of calories from fat (an amount that was once thought to be risky). A few years later, research on high-protein plans found that the higher amounts of fat in these diets didn't raise the risk of heart disease; in some studies, eating more fat actually lowered certain risk factors like cholesterol and artery inflammation.

Some newer studies even show that saturated fat may not be as bad as initially suspected. Certain foods that are higher in saturated fats, such as dark chocolate and eggs, have other healthy qualities like antioxidants, vitamins, and minerals that can enhance your diet.

One reason dieters benefit from adding healthy fat to their diets is that it tastes better, and it's more satisfying than simple carbohydrates. So go ahead and make more room in your weight-loss plan for avocados, eggs, olive oil, walnuts, oily fish like salmon, and lean cuts of beef. There's absolutely no reason why you can't eat well and still reach your goal weight.

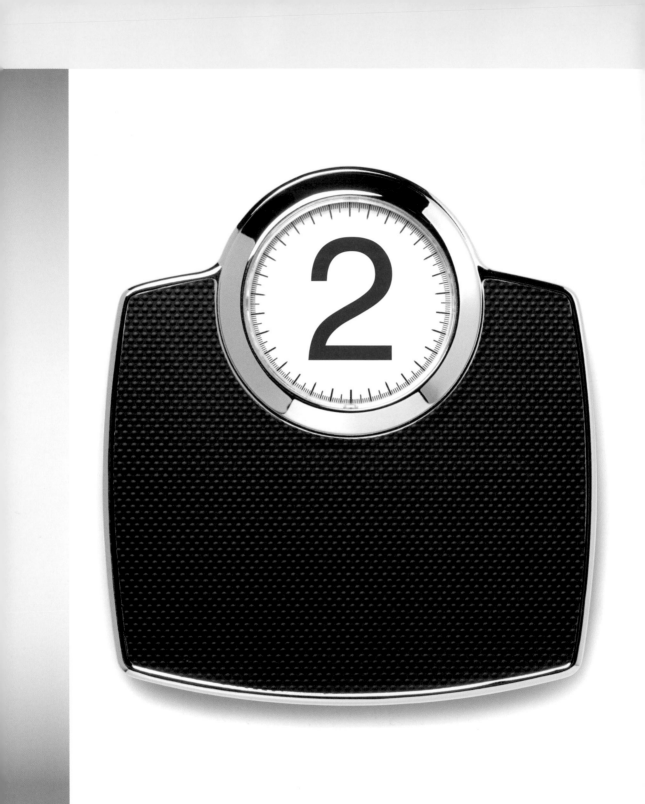

THE ZONE. ATKINS. DUKAN. WEIGHT WATCHERS. ORNISH.** All of these diets promote themselves as healthy ways to eat. Each plan comes with promises of dramatic weight loss. Yet they won't do you any good if you're gluten-sensitive. None of them takes into account the unique needs of the person who can't tolerate wheat, barley, rye, triticale, or anything that contains even a trace of gluten—a dizzying array of foods. Gluten is almost everywhere.

With the staggering increase in the number of people who respond poorly to gluten, more and more dieters are becoming frustrated with the alternatives and seeking out the only way of eating that will eliminate the source of their dietary troubles: They're going gluten free.

Just keep in mind that eating is supposed to make you feel good. When you sit down to a meal, the aftermath should not include gas, bloating, diarrhea, constipation, or nausea. Eating should make you feel energized, not headachy, fatigued, distracted, depressed, or awful.

For long-suffering gluten-sensitive people, this will come as a surprise. If you're in this group, you've no doubt spent a lifetime expecting and managing these unbearable symptoms. It's easy to assume that this is what life should be like: Eat, feel terrible, repeat. Gain weight, suffer achy joints, wrestle with migraines, and feel exhausted doing the most mundane activities.

The truth is that you don't have to live with pain and suffering. Change your diet, and those persistent, unpleasant symptoms will evaporate. You'll finally experience the gratification and satisfaction you should expect after replenishing your body.

Removing what is essentially a toxin from your diet will do wonders for your health. It's exactly that hope that drove you to purchase this book. What you may not realize is that there are other benefits to removing these grains from your diet, and altogether they add up to a far healthier way of living. Here are just a few.

Less Processed Food

One easy way to cut many sources of gluten out of your diet is to make your own meals at home rather than relying on packaged and prepared foods. As researchers probe the modern diet to find out why the way we eat causes us to gain weight, they repeatedly come back to one fundamental truth: Processed food, which is factory-produced; packed with salt, sugar, and artificial flavorings; stripped of vital nutrients; and often a source of gluten, equals disaster for the body. Despite the obvious downside of these foods, most diet plans allow you to use them in your daily meals. In fact, you'll find a lot of gluten-free processed foods. Some plans even produce their own processed meals for sale in your local grocery store.

The issue with these low-quality foodstuffs is that while they may temporarily fill you up, they actually leave your body starving for good nutrition. You feel hungry after a big meal because you're craving the missing vitamins and minerals, not to mention the phytonutrients, antioxidants, and other valuable disease-fighting substances in unprocessed foods.

Fast food falls into this category as well. You wouldn't believe how many chemicals and flavorings are pumped into the average burger from a fast food chain. The sodium and sugar content in the food you get is often astronomically high. This stuff has been tested and tinkered with in laboratories for decades until food scientists could arrive at a food that triggers extreme flavor sensations that keep the public wanting more. By cutting fast food out of your diet, you'll rediscover the true, satisfying, and pleasurable flavors of real food.

Plenty of Produce

Many popular diet plans promise quick and dramatic weight loss, but there are some that restrict fruits and vegetables, which are a key component of a healthy diet. An advantage to going gluten free over other diet plans is that it will force you to eat more produce.

Produce delivers plenty of valuable disease-fighting substances that can also help you lose weight. Dusky greens, vibrant oranges, and sweet tomatoes not only taste amazing, but they're also packed full of vital nutrients. Better yet, their calorie-to-nutrient ratio can't be beat. And this is the problem with many restrictive diet plans. Yes, you can lose weight, but only at the expense of a variety of fresh, colorful fruits and veggies. If you've ever tried one of these plans, you already know how wrong it feels to deny your body these valuable, tasty foods.

The Hidden Health Bonuses

One of the oddest aspects of going gluten free is that you're ridding your diet of foods that you've been taught are among the healthiest available. Wheat, barley, rye, and triticale contain vitamin E and plenty of fiber, and compose—in whole-grain form—a complete nutritional package. While giving up these grains may initially give you pause, there's research that suggests our digestive tracts aren't really set up to deal with these grains at all.

From an evolutionary perspective, farming practices are relatively new to humans. Our ancestors, who, after all, are the architects of our current digestive system, evolved eating primarily what they could scavenge from trees and bushes (fruits, vegetables, nuts, and seeds) and what they could hunt and kill (meat and fish). Research suggests that our digestive tract thrives while digesting these ancestral foods but can struggle when trying to process more recently developed agricultural products, such as—you guessed it—wheat, barley, rye, and triticale. And gluten seems to be the root of the trouble.

For those who have celiac disease or wheat allergy, the damage done to the gastrointestinal tract means many nutrients are not absorbed. Your ability to digest *all* foods, not just grains, can be compromised. In a world of easy access to cheap fast food, one of the side effects of malnutrition can be overeating. When the body is craving vital vitamins and minerals it's missing, it triggers the release of hormonal signals that stimulate hunger, researchers at the University of Chicago have found. Cleansing your diet of these gluten-containing grains can help ensure your body gleans the nutrients it craves from the foods you eat, and this can help you control your weight. But you may be surprised to learn that there are other benefits to cutting back on these grains.

• **Decreased hunger**: One of the challenges when dieting is recognizing when you're full. Some studies indicate that certain components in gluten can mess with the ability of leptin, a hormone that communicates between your stomach and your brain, to let your brain know you are full and to stop eating. Leptin resistance—when leptin isn't sending messages to your brain correctly—has been linked to an increased risk of becoming obese or overweight.

• **Fewer hormones**: One of the problems of our modern lifestyle is that we're exposed to too many hormones—especially xenoestrogens, which are found in pesticides, herbicides, and fungicides that factory farms use on crops, such as wheat, barley, rye, and triticale. These xenoestrogens can mimic the hormone estrogen, which may promote the retention of fat in the body.

• **Healthier thyroid:** To get soft, pillowy slices of bread, food makers rely on a chemical dough conditioner called potassium bromate. The problem is that this conditioner also happens to be an endocrine disruptor—in preliminary studies it has been shown to interrupt the flow of the body's natural hormones and has been linked to an increased risk of thyroid cancer. But long before it spurs tumor growth, the conditioner can slow down your thyroid. One of this gland's jobs is to regulate metabolism; as the gland's activity decreases, so does your metabolism. That equals fewer calories burned and more fat on your body.

• **Less starch**: Food scientists call a critical ingredient in bread—amylopectin A—the super starch. This sugar helps bread rise and become fluffy, but in your body it behaves just like white sugar: It dramatically raises blood sugar. That leads to inflammation and insulin resistance because your body must work extra hard to process all that sugar.

Why Gluten Free Is Nutritionally Healthy

A concern for people going gluten free is whether they'll get all the nutrients they need. The good news is that several studies have demonstrated that eating the full complement of gluten-free foods does in fact provide all the nutrients you need. Studies by Loren Cordain, Ph.D., one of the originators of the Paleo diet, which recommends avoiding all grains and is a loose way of going gluten free, has found that the diet can provide anywhere from double to 10 times the amount of your daily requirements for vitamins and minerals. You can rest assured that there's no reason to take supplements when you go gluten free.

Cutting out wheat, barley, rye, and triticale means you're also depriving yourself of some significant sources of fiber. Just remember that you'll be exploring a whole new world of gluten-free grains. From amaranth to teff, you'll discover that these whole grains, which are also rich in fiber, can make up for whatever you might be missing when you're eating gluten free. And don't forget that the extra fruit, vegetables, and seeds that are part of your regular eating repertoire also contain plenty of fiber.

What About All The Protein?

When you're gluten free, it's possible that more of your calories will come from protein. Don't be alarmed. In fact, you can take comfort in knowing that the protein content of your diet is trending upward. The latest research suggests that if you want to lose weight, adding more lean beef, poultry, and fish into your meals is exactly what you need. It may be exactly what you've been missing.

In 2009, researchers at the University of Illinois and Penn State University conducted a 12-month university study of 130 people looking to shed some pounds. Half of them followed a high-carbohydrate, low-fat, low-protein diet inspired by the USDA food pyramid. The rest followed a diet moderately high in protein, about what you'll get on the *10 Pounds Off Gluten-Free Diet*. The researchers taught the volunteers to shop and prepare meals based on the plan they were following, then tracked the dieters through an active four-month weight-loss phase and then for an additional eight months while the dieters attempted to maintain their loss.

After a year, the high-protein group had lost 23 percent more weight—and kept it off—than the low-fat dieters. It was a clear win for high-protein eating, but the news was even better than at first blush. When the researchers analyzed the volunteers' bodies, they discovered that the high-protein group had lost 22 percent more body fat during the four-month weight-loss phase than the low-fat group.

Even more remarkable, the high-protein group continued to shed body fat through the eight-month maintenance phase. At the end of 12 months, the high-protein dieters had lost 38 percent more body fat than the low-fat group. How could this happen? The researchers believe that the boost in filling, slow-to-digest protein helped control hunger and reduce snacking. The additional protein created an environment in the body that encouraged the growth of muscle; because muscles burn more calories than fat, the diet created a self-sustaining weight maintenance process, the researchers theorize.

The findings underline the true value of eating more protein: Yes, you'll lose more weight because you'll feel fuller than you would on a high-carbohydrate plan. But you'll also preferentially shed unhealthy and unsightly body fat while preserving your calorie-burning muscles. By the way, the other finding from the study was that, at year's end, more than half of the low-fat group had dropped out of the study, while two-thirds of the high-protein dieters were still going strong. The bottom line: Going gluten free will not only help heal your gut; it may be the quickest, most effective, and easiest way to drop weight.

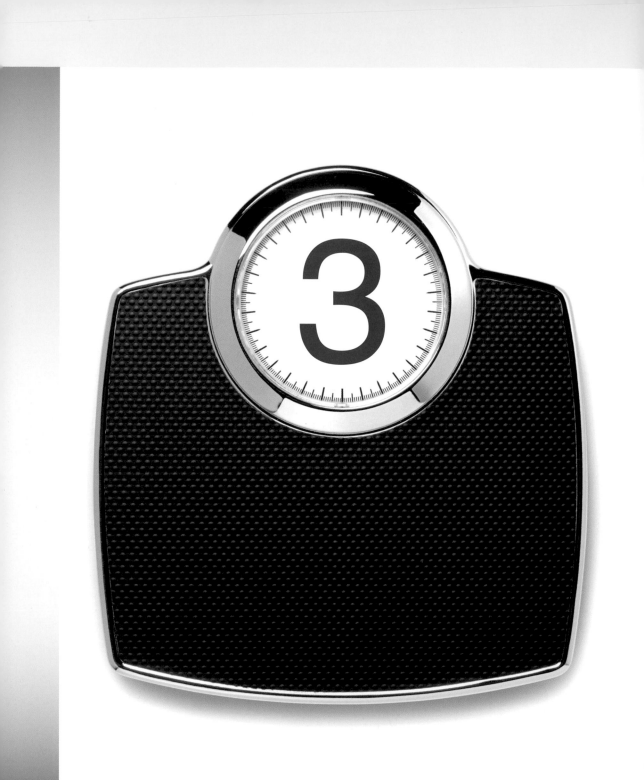

THE NUTS AND BOLTS OF GOING GLUTEN FREE

DEPENDING ON YOUR LEVEL OF SENSITIVITY, the effects of exposure to even a little gluten can be severe. As a result, you'll need to use vigilance in avoiding foods that contain it. You probably already know it's in breads, pastas, crackers, and cereals made with wheat, barley, rye, or triticale. But thanks to gluten's texture and binding qualities, it also turns up in stocks, sauces, salad dressings, chips, spices, deli meats, fast food, and candy. You can even find it in beauty products.

To eliminate gluten from your life, you'll have to develop your detecting skills. You'll need to read labels closely and learn to watch for the ingredients that may contain gluten—it's usually in one of the ingredients, not listed on its own. You may even need to call the manufacturer to verify that a product is gluten free. Oats, for example, don't contain gluten, but they're often processed on the same equipment as gluten-containing grain and therefore can be cross-contaminated.

Don't despair, though: Numerous gluten-free products are available in stores and online—from baking mixes and flours to pizza doughs and pastas—and new products are added all the time. While many gluten-free products, like sauces and condiments, can be used interchangeably with their gluten-containing counterparts, some need to be handled differently. These include primarily products that would normally contain gluten (breads, pastas, baking mixes, desserts) but have been made with gluten-free ingredients. When cooking with such foods, be sure to reference the packages and use the cooking instructions specified for that product. Various brands of the same product can also act differently based on the mix of ingredients and the amounts of each ingredient they contain, so a procedure and cooking time that worked perfectly for quinoa pasta won't always work for rice pasta, and one pancake mix may have a different texture than another. Follow the package directions and our instructions in the recipes closely for the best results.

Of course, there's another way to avoid gluten: If you make the effort to prepare most of your food at home using fresh ingredients, you'll have the most control over what goes into your body. Fresh ingredients, like fresh produce, lean protein, and gluten-free whole grains, are healthier choices than packaged foods, even if they are gluten free. Once you've stocked your kitchen, you'll be able to prepare gluten-free meals without a worry.

On the following pages we'll guide you to the foods you can keep on hand to make delicious meals that are also gluten free. And in some cases, when you need to make substitutions, we'll explain how to make gluten free work for baking and other uses.

Foods You Can Eat

Although you might feel like you're entering a strange new world of strict limitations when you go gluten free, there are a surprising number of familiar foods still on the menu. The following foods can fit into your new way of eating with ease. Just remember: If you want to trust that these foods are gluten-free, you must buy them unseasoned, unprocessed, and unprepared—in their most natural state, in other words.

Beans	Meat
Dairy	Nuts and seeds
Eggs	Poultry
Fish	Shellfish
Fruits	Vegetables

Good Grains and Starches

There are numerous grains that don't contain gluten. And yes, it *is* possible to bake and still be gluten free. Below is a list of the safe grains.

Amaranth	Polenta
Arrowroot	Potato flour
Buckwheat	Potato starch
Corn	Potatoes
Cornstarch	Quinoa
Grits	Rice
Hominy	Sorghum
Millet	Tapioca
Montina™ (Indian ricegrass)	Teff
Oats*	

*Choose oats marked "certified gluten free" since there's a risk of cross-contamination.

Below you'll find a list of alternative flours you can experiment with to help create your favorite baked goods.

ALMOND MEAL FLOUR: Ground from whole, blanched almonds, this high-protein flour adds a superb texture and nutty flavor.
Shelf life: Store in an airtight container in refrigerator or freezer up to six months.
Best for: biscuits, pancakes, waffles, muffins, cookies, piecrusts, and cakes

AMARANTH FLOUR: This flour is made from amaranth seeds that have been ground into dense flour.
Shelf life: Store in an airtight container in refrigerator or freezer up to six months.
Best for: pancakes, crepes, muffins, breads, crackers, and cookies

ARROWROOT STARCH: This tasteless white flour derived from the base of the arrowroot plant is an excellent substitute for cornstarch in baked goods.
Shelf life: Store in an airtight container in a cool, dry place up to six months.
Best for: breads and biscuits

BROWN RICE FLOUR: This flour is a staple in gluten-free baking. It's dense with a grainy texture and nutty flavor and works best when blended with other gluten-free flours.
Shelf life: Store in an airtight container in refrigerator up to six months.
Best for: pancakes, waffles, crepes, piecrusts, biscuits, muffins, cookies, cakes, and pastries

BUCKWHEAT FLOUR: Despite its name, buckwheat flour doesn't contain any wheat. Rather, buckwheat is a grain-like seed that's ground into flour. It has an earthy, nutty flavor.

Shelf life: Store in an airtight container in refrigerator up to six months or in freezer up to one year.

Best for: breakfast cereals, breads, pancakes, and waffles

COCONUT FLOUR: Coconut flour is ground from dried, defatted coconut meat. It works best when combined with other gluten-free flours.

Shelf life: Store in an airtight container in refrigerator or freezer up to six months.

Best for: pancakes, cakes, muffins, and breads

CORN FLOUR: Corn flour is ground from whole corn kernels into a texture much finer than traditional cornmeal. Variations include masa harina, which is ground from white or yellow corn, and harinilla, which is ground blue corn.

Shelf life: Store in an airtight container in refrigerator up to six months or freezer up to one year.

Best for: breads, pizza crusts, muffins, pancakes, cakes, and tortillas

CORNMEAL: Ground from whole corn kernels into a gritty meal, cornmeal is much coarser than corn flour. It adds a sweet, nutty flavor to a variety of baked goods.

Shelf life: Store in an airtight container in a cool, dry place up to two months or in refrigerator up to six months.

Best for: breads, muffins, pizza crusts, and tortillas

CORNSTARCH: This is a flavorless, fine white powder that adds airiness to gluten-free baked goods. It works best when blended with other gluten-free flours.

Shelf life: Store in an airtight container in a cool, dry place up to two years.

Best for: pancakes, muffins, biscuits, breads, and cakes

FLAXSEED MEAL: Made from flax-seeds that have been ground into a dense flour, flaxseed meal works best when blended with other gluten-free flours.
Shelf life: Store in an airtight container in refrigerator up to six months or freezer up to one year.
Best for: pancakes, waffles, muffins, and breads

HAZELNUT FLOUR: This sweet, tawny, high-protein flour is made from finely ground hazelnuts.
Shelf life: Store in an airtight container in refrigerator up to six months.
Best for: breads, muffins, cookies, and cakes

MILLET FLOUR: This highly nutritious flour is ground from millet grains. It imparts a sweet and nutty flavor to baked goods and also gives them a crumbly texture.
Shelf life: Store in an airtight container in refrigerator up to six months.
Best for: breads and muffins

OAT FLOUR: Oat flour is made from very finely ground oats. It adds a robust taste and hearty texture to baked goods. To avoid cross-contamination, purchase oat flour that's certified gluten free.
Shelf life: Store in an airtight container in a cool, dry place up to three months or in refrigerator or freezer up to six months.
Best for: muffins, breads, cookies, and cakes

INGREDIENT TIP

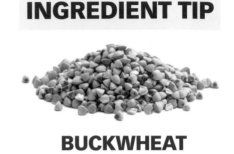

BUCKWHEAT

BUCKWHEAT is a misleading term. It's not wheat but rather a naturally gluten-free seed. It's a whole grain, which carries many health benefits such as helping to reduce blood cholesterol levels, and is less starchy and higher in fiber than gluten-free corn or rice.

QUINOA FLOUR: Ground from seeds, quinoa flour is a nutritious, high-protein flour that has a slightly nutty flavor.
Shelf life: Store in an airtight container in refrigerator up to six months.
Best for: biscuits, muffins, cookies, breads, and cakes

SORGHUM FLOUR: Sorghum flour is ground from a high-protein, high-fiber cereal grain. It is heavy and should be blended with lighter, starchier flours.
Shelf life: Store in an airtight container up to three months, in refrigerator up to six months, or in freezer up to one year.
Best for: muffins, pancakes, biscuits, cookies, cakes, and breads

SWEET POTATO FLOUR: When added to baked goods, sweet potato flour helps them retain moisture while enhancing nutrition and adding richness.
Shelf life: Store in an airtight container in a cool, dry place up to one year.
Best for: pancakes, crepes, breads, and muffins

TAPIOCA FLOUR (STARCH): A light, powdery, tasteless flour, tapioca flour adds body and chewy texture to baked goods. It works best when combined with other gluten-free flours.
Shelf life: Store in an airtight container in a cool, dry place up to two years.
Best for: pancakes, muffins, biscuits, cookies, cakes, and breads

TEFF FLOUR: This finely textured flour is milled from a grain named teff.
Shelf life: Store in an airtight container in refrigerator up to six months.
Best for: pancakes, muffins, breads, and tortillas

WHITE RICE FLOUR: This flour is derived from white rice that has been ground into a light, powdery flour. It is a gluten-free baking staple. Use it interchangeably with brown rice flour.

Shelf life: Store in an airtight container in a cool, dry place up to one year.

Best for: pancakes, waffles, crepes, piecrusts, biscuits, muffins, cookies, brownies, cakes, and pastries

The "Maybe" Foods

These foods may be made with or without gluten, so it is important to read labels to find a safe version. By law, companies have to list wheat on the label if it is found in any ingredient, but you'll still want to double-check. For more information on where gluten may hide, see "Decoding Food Labels" on page 38.

Baked goods like bread, breadcrumbs, cakes, cookies, croutons, muffins, and piecrusts

Beer

Bouillon

Breading and coating mixes

Broth (all varieties)

Candy

Cereal

Coated popcorn and chips

Corn tortillas

Crackers

Energy bars

Fast food

Flavored alcoholic drinks

Flavored or coated nuts and seeds

Flavored teas

Gravies, marinades, and sauces

Hoisin sauce

Licorice

Ice cream

Imitation seafood

Marinades

Multigrain rice and corn cakes

Oats (look for gluten-free oats)

Pastas

Pepperoni

Prepackaged convenience foods

Prepared icings and frostings

Prepared salsas

Processed foods

Processed meats (hot dogs, lunchmeat, and sausage)

Roasted nuts

Rotisserie chicken

Salad dressings

Sauces and gravies

Seasoned rice mixes

Seasoning mixes

Soups

Soy sauce

Spices (if there is no ingredient list on the label, then it contains only the pure spice)

Teriyaki sauce

Vegetables packaged with sauces

Worcestershire sauce

Yogurt (with granola)

INGREDIENT TIP

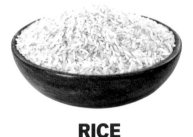

RICE

RICE can become an easy fall-back when you're going gluten free. You'll find it's used to make gluten-free pasta, baked goods, and cereals. But Consumer Reports found small but measurable amounts of arsenic in most rice products, and the organization warns against relying too heavily on rice-based substitutes.

Decoding Food Labels

Reading food labels is a must. Sometimes, the distinctions between gluten-free and gluten-containing foods aren't obvious until you read the label. Food companies manufacture their products differently, and the ingredients often vary from brand to brand. So it's vital to learn the names of ingredients that could cause concern if you see them on food labels. With practice, patience, and time, label reading will become second nature.

BARLEY: Barley appears on labels as malt, malt extract, malt flavoring, malt syrup, malt vinegar, barley malt flavoring, barley malt syrup, and brown rice syrup (which may be made with barley enzymes). All of these terms indicate the presence of gluten, and the item should be avoided.

CARAMEL COLOR: This ingredient, when manufactured in North America, is produced from corn and is gluten free.

HYDROLYZED VEGETABLE PROTEIN: This term is not used on a label. Instead, the label must specify the vegetable or grain, such as "hydrolyzed wheat protein," which is not gluten free, or "hydrolyzed soy protein," which is gluten free.

MALTODEXTRIN: This ingredient is made from corn, potato, or rice and should not be confused with the barley-containing ingredients known as malt or malt flavoring. If wheat was used, the label would have to say "wheat maltodextrin," "maltodextrin (wheat)," "dextrates," and "dextrimaltose." The term "dextrin" is rarely used on food labels.

MODIFIED FOOD STARCH: This ingredient can be made from wheat, but the label must say "wheat."

WHEAT STARCH: The starch is used as a binder and thickening agent in foods. If it is used as an ingredient, the label must say "wheat."

"I had no idea how life-changing it would be. It went beyond eating food. My body felt better."

Success Story:
Dorothy

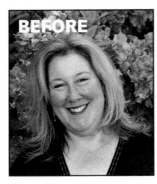

BEFORE

Age: 52

Height: 5'6"

**Weight before:
250**

**Weight after:
228**

Dorothy suffered from high blood pressure, internal inflammation, GI issues, swollen feet and ankles, and very low energy. Additionally, she was overweight. She never thought she could stick to a diet. When invited to participate in a 6-month gluten-free challenge, she decided to give it a try.

Focusing on eating healthier and accepting herself, Dorothy began to feel healthier and more confident. Her sweet tooth subsided and her hunger cravings decreased. Her blood pressure dropped and her swollen feet and ankles returned to normal. She learned to cook and planned her meals and snacks throughout her day. Most importantly, she had a support group and blogged about her experience. Dorothy saw the pounds shed and learned to love her body. "I had no idea how life-changing it would be. It went beyond eating food. My body felt better."

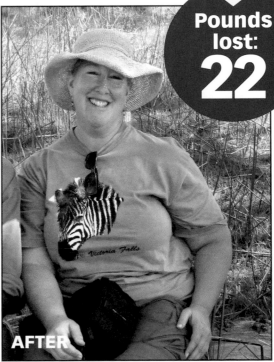

**Pounds
lost:
22**

AFTER

Foods to Avoid

The primary grains you need to avoid are wheat, barley, rye, triticale (a hybrid grain), and possibly oats (due to cross-contamination). But those are the primary forms of gluten. It can also turn up in other forms in foods, so refer to the following list when in doubt. Whether it's the primary ingredient or way down the list, the appearance of one of these items in the ingredients indicates that the food contains gluten.

Barley

Barley malt

Bran (oat, wheat)

Brewer's yeast

Bulgur

Cooking spray for baking (may contain wheat flour)

Couscous

Durum

Einkorn

Emmer

Farina

Farro

Flour containing wheat, barley, or rye or any of their derivatives

Graham flour

Hydrolyzed wheat protein

Kamut/khorasan wheat

Malted milk

Malt flavorings

Malt vinegar

Matzo

Meat, poultry, seafood, or vegetables that are breaded, floured, served with a sauce made from wheat, or marinated in a wheat-based sauce such as soy or teriyaki

Rye

Seitan

Semolina

Spelt

Triticale

Wheat

Wheat germ

Wheat starch

Wheatberries

Although there isn't much of a gluten concern with soda and diet soda, you'll still want to limit or eliminate your intake. Soda of course is loaded with sugar and no friend to weight-loss efforts. While diet soda and artificial sweeteners might seem harmless and a good alternative, they're not. Any savings they offer are illusory.

When Harvard researchers tracked people who primarily drank artificially sweetened beverages, they discovered that the diet soda drinkers gained more weight than people who drank regular soda (though both groups put on pounds). Back in the lab, the researchers discovered that when rats are given artificial sweeteners they actually eat more food than rats that get real sugar, possibly because calorie sensors in the gut and brain expect to gain energy from such a sweet taste. When the calories fail to turn up, these sensors prompted the rats to overeat to compensate.

The saccharin taste of these artificial sweeteners—which taste as much as a hundred times sweeter than sugar—presents another problem, say experts. We're training our taste buds to expect extreme flavors, and simple, good, sweet food like fruit pales in comparison. We end up shunning it in favor of the sensationally sweet foods.

Cut out the diet soda—and the regular soda. You'll miss them initially, but you can replace the drink with seltzer sweetened with a squeeze of lemon or lime. Within a week or two your taste buds will have recalibrated themselves, and you'll get more pleasure from a truly healthy (and weight-loss–friendly) diet.

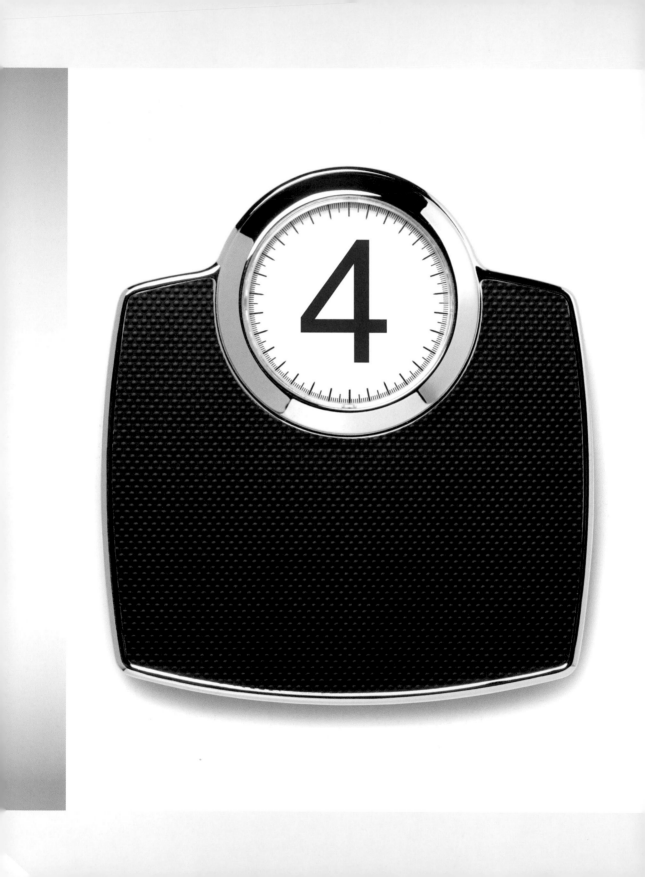

PUTTING YOUR GLUTEN-FREE DIET INTO ACTION

NOW THAT YOU KNOW what you can and can't eat on your diet, it's time to clear out your kitchen. The easiest way to do this is if your entire household is going gluten free—then you can just donate or toss all the offending foods. However, it's unlikely this will be possible unless you live alone or with one other person.

If you're the only person making the gluten-free leap, try designating certain areas of your pantry, freezer, food shelves, and refrigerator as gluten-free zones.

What about alcohol?
You'll be happy to
hear that most forms
are okay. Beer is
definitely a no-no
(unless it's labeled
gluten free), but
wine, whiskey, gin,
vodka, brandy, rum,
and tequila are all
gluten free!

Now take a hard look at the food in your house. This will
be good practice for future shopping trips. Analyze the
ingredient labels for signs of wheat, barley, and rye. Refer
back to the list of possible pseudonyms for gluten ingredients on page 38. Check the cereal boxes, the boxes of
"just add water" food products like macaroni and cheese,
and canned soups.

Finding the primary offenders is easy: You can toss the
bread and bagels; white and wheat flour; barley; bran;
bulgur; malt vinegar; breaded meat, poultry, or fish; and
the wheat germ as well as the crackers and cookies. And
while you're at it, clear out the sodas and beer. If the food
is unopened, you might be able to donate it. The rest a neighbor or relative
might be open to taking.

GLUTEN-FREE SPICES

Once you've cleared the shelves, take a look at Chapter 6 on page 62 for a
shopping list of gluten-free basics that you'll want to stock your cabinets
with. One area you'll want to be sure is complete is your spice rack. Now
that you'll be preparing more of your meals from scratch, spices are your
ally. As long as there's only one ingredient on the label of the spice jar, it
should be gluten free—but beware that some mixes may contain gluten.
Here's a list of spices to keep on hand:

Bay leaves	Coriander	Mint
Black pepper	Crushed red pepper flakes	Oregano
Cayenne pepper	Cumin	Paprika
Cinnamon	Garlic powder	Rosemary
Cloves	Ginger	Salt
Cocoa	Ground mustard	Thyme

You may want to consider planting an herb garden as well, which allows you to have fresh herbs on hand at all times without having to run out to the grocery store. You can even grow herbs indoors with new kits on the market, and there's nothing like fresh basil, cilantro, rosemary, and thyme to liven up a dish.

Gluten-Free Tools

Here's a list of the tools and equipment you might need to create delicious gluten-free meals at home. A note on kitchen safety: If you also prepare foods that contain gluten in your kitchen, preventing cross-contamination is key. You'll need to thoroughly clean dishes, counters, cooking surfaces, and kitchen utensils and appliances after any of them have come into contact with foods containing gluten. (In a perfect world, separate appliances and small wares, such as cutting boards and flour sifters, would be best.) You probably have plenty of kitchen utensils and appliances on hand, but peruse this list to see if you're missing anything. These items aren't essential, but they will make preparing meals for your new eating plan much simpler.

KITCHEN SCALE Because each person scoops flour into a measuring cup differently, a kitchen scale is ideal because it allows for accurate measurements every time. A digital scale is the easiest to use, but a top-loading or hanging scale will also work.

LIQUID MEASURING CUPS Liquid measuring cups are usually made of glass, plastic, or stainless steel and are used to measure ingredients such as water, juices, milks, oils, and honey.

DRY MEASURING CUPS Dry measuring cups are usually made of plastic or stainless steel and are used to measure ingredients like flour, sugar, dried fruits, and nuts.

MEASURING SPOONS Measuring spoons are usually made of plastic, metal, or porcelain. They're used to measure smaller amounts of ingredients, such as spices, herbs, sugar, vanilla extract, baking soda, baking powder, xanthan gum, and yeast.

GRATER AND ZESTER These two essential pieces of equipment come in handy for grating a variety of ingredients like cheese, carrots, and zucchini. They are also needed to achieve the right texture, weight, and consistency when grating nutmeg or citrus rinds, which add flavor to baked goods.

HIGH-QUALITY KNIVES A sharp knife is a blessing in the kitchen. It turns a prep job from a chore to a pleasure. And the sharper the better: Dull knives are far more likely to slip and slice your finger than sharp ones. (So consider a high-quality sharpener to help maintain your knives' edges.)

SPIRALIZER This device can do wonderful things with vegetables to help them fill in for the grain foods you may be missing. You can turn squash, carrots, and other firm veggies into noodles for a pasta substitute, for noodles in a soup, or for an interesting textured filling in a lettuce wrap.

DIGITAL THERMOMETER When you'll be preparing lots of meat, this is an invaluable tool. The digital versions can give you a much faster read. Some include the option of leaving the sensor in the meat as it cooks in the oven or on the grill while the readout monitor sits on the counter so you know exactly when your meat is at the proper temperature.

EGG POACHERS Eggs are an excellent source of nutrition for gluten-free eaters. You may tire of fried eggs, scrambled eggs, and hard-cooked eggs, which is why having egg poachers on hand can help you keep your break-fasts feeling fresh. You can get silicone cups that float in boiling water, allowing you to poach eggs to perfection. Mix them with some quick-braised greens for a healthy start to your day.

8-INCH CAST-IRON SKILLET You'll find this skillet is perfect for whipping up a quick gluten-free breakfast, such as eggs and uncured ham. These pans typically come preseasoned, so all you have to do is be sure to keep it in shape. Use vegetable oil, canola oil, olive oil, or butter when you cook; rinse the skillet—no soap!—right after you finish and use a dishwashing brush to knock off the food scraps. Thoroughly dry the pan and smear a little of your cooking oil all over the top and bottom. Keep the skillet in a dry place that's handy. Food simply tastes better when made in these pans, and the care is so simple you'll wonder why you ever bothered with so-called nonstick cookware!

10- OR 12-INCH CAST-IRON SKILLET This larger skillet will be your go-to pan for cooking most of your dinner meals, whether it's searing steaks, crisping roasts that you'll finish in the oven (the great advantage of these pans is they can easily go from the stove top to the oven and back again), or whipping up stir-fries. Unlike most cookware, these hardy pans improve with age; their seasoning adds flavor to everything you cook. If you want to keep things simple, opt for this larger pan. You can use it to prepare smaller meals and breakfasts, too.

BAKING SHEETS Roasting vegetables like cauliflower, asparagus, and broccoli with olive oil, garlic, and pepper turns them into gourmet delights. Kale chips can stand in for any grain alternative. But to pull these dishes off with ease and panache, you'll need a good supply of baking sheets. Keep your cleanup quick and easy by lining the sheets with aluminum foil or parchment paper before baking.

TIP

Keep your kitchen safe. Cross-contamination with gluten can occur in food-processing plants—but it can also happen in your kitchen. If you're the only one going gluten free in your home, you'll want to keep duplicates of jarred foods that everyone eats, like peanut butter, and label the one that's yours. Otherwise, the knife used to spread peanut butter on bread will transfer small amounts of gluten to the jar.

SEPARATE CUTTING BOARDS If you prepare foods that contain gluten, it would be smart to purchase a cutting board specifically for prepping gluten-free ingredients. Cutting boards made of wood or bamboo have porous surfaces, which are hard to clean and have nooks and crannies where gluten can adhere.

STOCKPOT If you aren't making your own stock, now's the time to start. The store-bought stuff can be high in sodium and usually contains gluten. Drop a leftover chicken carcass or beef bones, roughly chopped onions, celery, carrots, and your choice of spices into a stockpot full of water, and let it simmer for an hour or so—you'll have the best stock you've ever had. Choose a big pot—20 quarts isn't too big. (You can always freeze your left-over stock.) If you don't have time to make your own, be sure to purchase reduced-sodium varieties of store-bought stock or broth.

MIXERS The three most popular baking mixers include the stand mixer, hand mixer, and immersion blender (also called a stick mixer). Electric mixers are designed to do the work for you and ensure that all the ingredients get mixed evenly and uniformly. They also have different speeds that allow you to whip delicate ingredients such as egg whites or thick ingredients such as brownie batter or marshmallows. A hand mixer or immersion blender is ideal for smaller jobs that don't involve mixing heavy batters or doughs.

FOOD PROCESSOR The food processor is a must-have, multitasking tool vital for every kitchen. It slices, chops, shreds, purees, grinds, and mixes a variety of ingredients—it is the most versatile piece of equipment in the kitchen and can be a huge time-saver when prepping ingredients.

BLENDER A blender is used to mix, blend, or emulsify food. It is great for pureeing fruit for pie fillings or toppings or blending smoothies; bean dips; or batters for pancakes, crepes, or waffles.

IMMERSION BLENDER This will come in handy morning, noon, and night. You can use it to easily puree soups or mix sauces and salad dressings.

SLOW COOKER The simplest way to save yourself time at the end of the day is to make dinner in the morning. Throw a bunch of fresh ingredients into your cooker along with broth and some bay leaves before you leave for work. Voilà: At the end of the day your dinner is ready and the house will smell wonderful.

GOOD STORAGE CONTAINERS Prepare double or triple batches of your favorite meals and freeze the leftovers in high-quality, freezer-durable containers. That's one or more meals you won't have to prepare down the road!

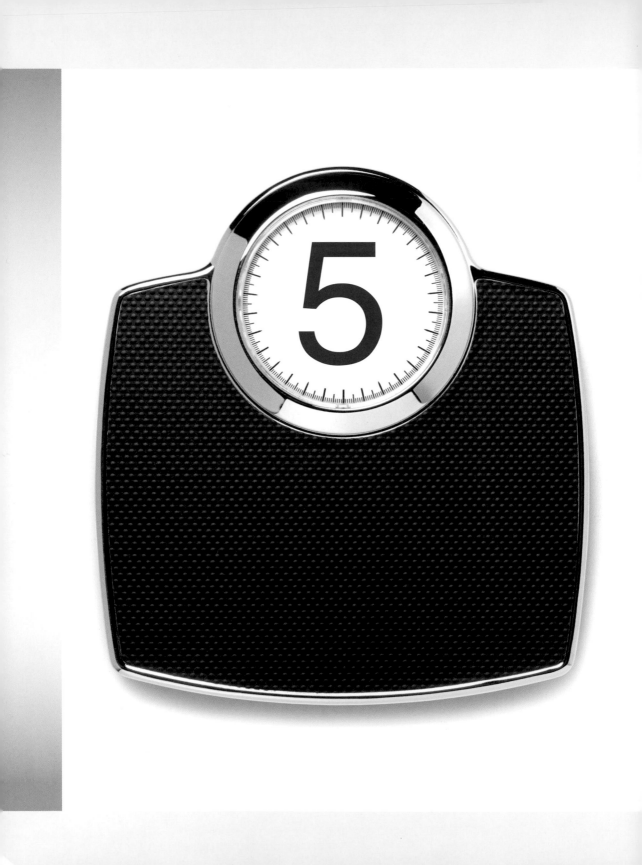

TAKE THE GLUTEN-FREE DIET CHALLENGE

ARE YOU READY TO DIVE IN? Your kitchen is prepared, you have the food you need, and more importantly, you've eliminated the foods you need to avoid. Now it's time to take the challenge. On the following pages there are four weeks of food plans that will help you lose at least the 10 pounds you want to drop and control any symptoms you might be having. You'll also feel better, especially if you add the exercise component from Chapter 12.

WEEK 1

	BREAKFAST	LUNCH	DINNER
MONDAY	**Mixed Berry Muffins** (pg. 83)	**Spicy-Sweet Chicken Lettuce Cups** (pg. 100)	**Salsa Flounder** (pg. 108)
TUESDAY	**Peppery Potato Omelet** (pg. 69)	**Portobello and Black Bean Quesadillas** (pg. 103)	**Cast-Iron Burgers** (pg. 118)
WEDNESDAY	**Sunflower Granola** (pg. 75)	**Pork Wraps with Fresh Tomatillo Salsa** (pg. 98)	**Citrus-Herb Chicken** (pg. 124)
THURSDAY	**Mexican Chorizo Hash** (pg. 73)	**Broccoli-Cheese Soup** (pg. 104)	**Roasted Pork Tenderloin Tacos** (pg. 119)
FRIDAY	**Quinoa with Strawberries and Buttermilk** (pg. 77)	**Warm Brown Rice and Chickpea Salad with Cherries and Goat Cheese** (pg. 92)	**Five-Bean Chili** (pg. 135)
SATURDAY	**Mushroom Frittata** (pg. 70)	**Salmon Salad on Arugula** (pg. 89)	**Three-Cheese Baked Penne** (pg. 140)
SUNDAY	**Oatmeal Pancakes** (pg. 80)	**Blueberry Chicken Salad** (pg. 94)	**Vegetarian Lasagna** (pg. 139)

WEEK 2

	BREAKFAST	LUNCH	DINNER
MONDAY	Breakfast Quinoa (pg. 79)	Tuna-Pecan Salad Sandwiches (pg. 94)	Greek-Style Chicken Breasts (pg. 129)
TUESDAY	Mexican Chorizo Hash (pg. 73)	Roasted Carrot, Chicken, and Grape Quinoa Bowl (pg. 93)	Pasta Carbonara Florentine (pg. 143)
WEDNESDAY	Savory Buckwheat with Tomato, Cheddar, and Bacon (pg. 77)	Banh Mi–Style Roast Beef Sandwiches (pg. 97)	Sausage Pizza (pg. 138)
THURSDAY	Vanilla Amaranth with Peach Compote (pg. 76)	Chicken-Olive Quesadillas (pg. 102)	Pork Tenderloin and Cannellini Beans (pg. 121)
FRIDAY	Pecan-Oatmeal Waffles (pg. 82)	Spicy Steak Lettuce Wraps (pg. 95)	Chicken with Turnips and Pomegranate Sauce (pg. 126)
SATURDAY	Zucchini and Red Pepper Frittata (pg. 71)	Black Bean Soup (pg. 105)	Cedar Plank Salmon with Tomato Salsa (pg. 110)
SUNDAY	Cheesy Hash Brown Casserole (pg. 74)	Spicy Chicken Sandwiches (pg. 99)	Tomato-Basil Pasta with Asiago (pg. 141)

	BREAKFAST	LUNCH	DINNER
MONDAY	Pumpkinseed-Almond Granola (pg. 75)	Portobello and Black Bean Quesadillas (pg. 103)	Shredded Chicken Tacos with Tomatoes and Grilled Corn (pg. 127)
TUESDAY	Mexican Chorizo Hash (pg. 73)	Banh Mi–Style Roast Beef Sandwiches (pg. 97)	Tilapia Veracruz (pg. 113)
WEDNESDAY	Quinoa with Strawberries and Buttermilk (pg. 77)	Broccoli-Cheese Soup (pg. 104)	Slow-Cooker Brisket (pg. 117)
THURSDAY	Peppery Potato Omelet (pg. 69)	Pork Wraps with Fresh Tomatillo Salsa (pg. 98)	Saffron Rice with Tilapia and Shrimp (pg. 111)
FRIDAY	Blueberry-Almond Oatmeal Pancakes (pg. 81)	Spicy-Sweet Chicken Lettuce Cups (pg. 100)	Stuffed Poblanos (pg. 137)
SATURDAY	Breakfast Quinoa (pg. 79)	Roasted Carrot, Chicken, and Grape Quinoa Bowl (pg. 93)	Pork Tenderloin with Roasted Cherries and Shallots (pg. 123)
SUNDAY	Zucchini and Red Pepper Frittata (pg. 71)	Spicy Bean and Quinoa Salad with "Mole" Vinaigrette (pg. 90)	Braised Chicken with Honey-Lemon Leeks (pg. 131)

	BREAKFAST	LUNCH	DINNER
MONDAY	Cinnamon, Apple, and Oat Scones (pg. 84)	Blueberry Chicken Salad (pg. 94)	Seared Scallops with Snap Peas and Pancetta (pg. 115)
TUESDAY	Savory Buckwheat with Tomato, Cheddar, and Bacon (pg. 77)	Tuna-Pecan Salad Sandwiches (pg. 94)	Pasta with Roasted Red Pepper and Cream Sauce (pg. 142)
WEDNESDAY	Sunflower Granola (pg. 75)	Warm Brown Rice and Chickpea Salad with Cherries and Goat Cheese (pg. 92)	Chicken Verde Enchiladas (pg. 130)
THURSDAY	Mushroom Frittata (pg. 70)	Black Bean Soup (pg. 105)	Grilled Chicken Thighs with Cilantro-Mint Chutney (pg. 132)
FRIDAY	Mixed Berry Muffins (pg. 83)	Salmon Salad on Arugula (pg. 89)	Sautéed Tilapia Tacos with Grilled Peppers and Onion (pg. 114)
SATURDAY	Vanilla Amaranth with Peach Compote (pg. 76)	Chicken-Olive Quesadillas (pg. 102)	Dijon-Herb Chicken Thighs (pg. 134)
SUNDAY	Cheesy Hash Brown Casserole (pg. 74)	Spicy Steak Lettuce Wraps (pg. 95)	Asian Rice with Shrimp and Snow Peas (pg. 116)

Snacks

There are recipes for snacks (check out Edamame Crunch, pg. 150, Lemon-Parmesan Popcorn, pg. 151, and Roasted Garlic and Chive Dip, pg. 146), but for the most part, you'll want to experiment to find the snacks that work best in terms of filling you up and satisfying your cravings. Here are some other ideas you can experiment with:

Fresh fruit	Gluten-free cereal
Dried fruit	Gluten-free tortilla chips
Raw vegetables	Nuts or seeds
Guacamole	Olives
Hummus	Hard-cooked egg
Peanut butter	String cheese
Gluten-free crackers	Greek yogurt
Gluten-free energy bars	

TIP

Go with what works.
If you find a break-fast that works for your taste buds, time, and budget, feel free to stick with that. Same with lunch, although for dinner and snacks, you may want to try the suggestions in the plan so that you'll have a chance to experience different flavors and preparations.

Dessert

Pleasing your sweet tooth is easier than you might think when you're going gluten free. You'll find plenty of dessert options in Chapter 11 (pg. 164). One tip to remember is that you can use arrowroot flour to thicken dessert sauces (and regular sauces as well), though you'll want to use cornstarch if you're making a dairy-based sauce. When you don't have time to prepare a special dessert, look for gluten-free dark chocolate—stick to a square at a time to satisfy your sweets craving.

Eating Out Gluten Free

One of the easy ways to run into trouble when trying to stay gluten free is eating out. You may have noticed, though, that more and more restaurants are offering gluten-free entrées. However, if you're really sensitive, you'll have to verify that the food is prepared with separate pans and utensils to avoid cross-contamination. The following tips can help you navigate most menus and restaurants with ease.

- **Check out the menu online before you go**. With a little planning you can figure out where you'll eat and what you'll have before you leave the house. If you find that your destination offers gluten-free options, give the restaurant a call (just not during mealtime rush!) and query the staff about how the food is prepared.
- **Get to know your server/chef.** If you're eating out near your place of work, you probably have two or three places you go regularly. Don't hesitate to ask questions about how the food is prepared to make sure it conforms to your new diet.
- **Let the waitstaff know that you're gluten sensitive**. Most restaurants are ready to accommodate people who are gluten intolerant. If the staff seems unclear what that means, briefly explain which ingredients are off-limits for you.
- **Be flexible**. You might find that the restaurant is out of the dish you planned to order or that the staff can't satisfactorily answer your questions. Pack some gluten-free snacks just in case. You could also order a plate of fresh vegetables to nosh on while your companions eat.

TIP

Ask your waiter.
It's okay to ask the waitstaff detailed questions about how food is prepared. Here are a few sample questions to tease out information:

- Are the French fries coated with flour?
- Are artificial bacon bits or other meat substitutes used on potato skins and salads?
- Does the salad dressing contain wheat or flour?
- Does the soup contain flour or barley?

Visit celiac.org for even more eating-out tips.

Eating Gluten Free on the Run

While preparing a beautiful meal and cooking more at home are the easiest ways to stay gluten free, the pressures of modern life often get in the way. Here are some ideas for quick breakfasts and lunches.

HARD-COOKED EGGS This is a simple, nutritious, and fast gluten-free breakfast. Pair it with some fresh fruit or kale chips, and you can start your day with a solid blast of nutrients and protein.

SMOOTHIE Throw some Greek yogurt, frozen berries, pineapple, mango, and ice into a blender for a smoothie that you can drink on your way to work and that will get you through your morning.

BARS AND MUFFINS You can find gluten-free breakfast muffins and energy bars at your local grocer. You can also make your own (so you can control the sugar). Check out the Mixed Berry Muffins (pg. 83), Cinnamon, Apple, and Oat Scones (pg. 84), Almond-Date Bars (pg. 175), and Maple-Pecan Bars (pg. 176).

TRAIL MIX Keep a plastic container full of your favorite roasted, unsalted nuts and dried fruit. Throw in some coconut flakes for variety.

BELL PEPPER OR CABBAGE SANDWICHES Slice bell pepper into wide, flat slabs, or peel off and wash sturdy, broad cabbage leaves to make sandwiches with sliced turkey, pitted olives, and the greens of your choice.

VEGGIES AND DIP Bring pieces of carrot, celery, broccoli, and cauliflower to dip in nut butter, hummus, or guacamole.

Traveling Gluten Free

When you're on the road, avoiding gluten can get a lot more difficult. One easy way to cover yourself is to pack a lot of snacks—they'll get you through situations where finding a gluten-free option may be tough. Here are some other tricks to keep in mind.

- **Find a gluten-free-friendly restaurant first**. If you can get a good breakfast to start your day, your battle is well on the way to being won.

- **Research local health/natural food stores**. If you don't want to waste time scanning grocery store shelves, you can get what you need here. The staff in these stores will be able to steer you to options and are more likely to be understanding and helpful about your sensitivity than the average chain grocery clerk.

- **Know your cuisines**. Mexican food can be gluten-free-friendly if you stick to the rice- or corn-based dishes. Watch out for the chips, flour tortillas, and anything that comes out of the deep fryer (no doubt the oil will also be used for gluten products). Thai cuisine is another great choice since the dishes typically rely on fish sauce (rather than the ubiquitous soy in Japanese and Chinese cuisines).

- **Pack plenty of options**. Let's face it, traveling adds plenty of challenges to remaining gluten free. So bring along a mini-pantry that can get you through the lean times, including bars, cereal, cookies, crackers, dried fruit, and nuts—pack as much as you can carry.

TIP

Cross-contamination concerns. When you're eating out, you should also ask your server about cross-contamination issues, like if there is a separate prep space for gluten-free foods, if separate utensils are used, and if they have a dedicated fryer (or change the frying oil) for gluten-free foods.

PART 2

100
GLUTEN-FREE
RECIPES

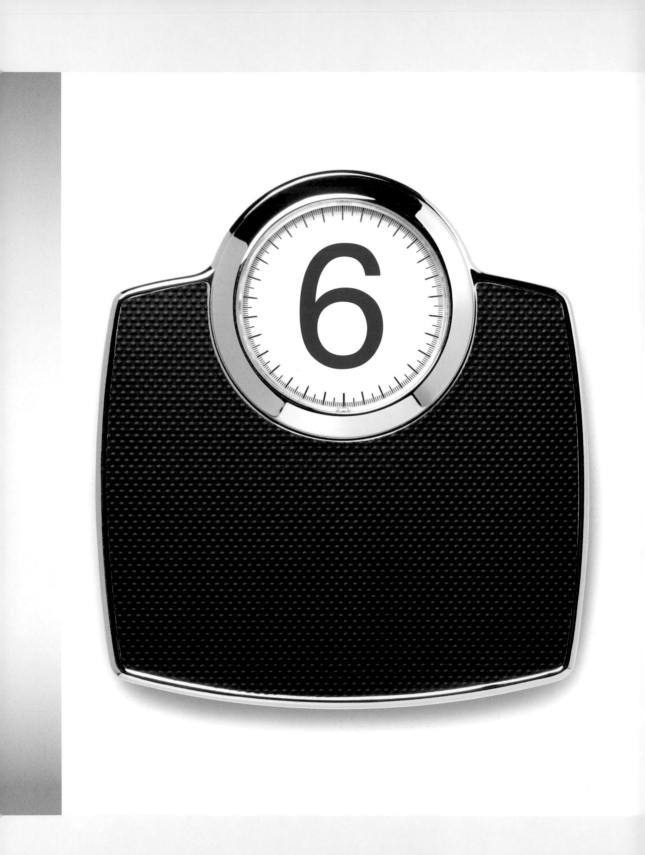

YOU MAY BE GOING GLUTEN **FREE,** but eating good food is still vitally important. Gluten free doesn't mean flavor free, so you'll find all of your favorite foods—from burgers and pastas to muffins and cakes—in these recipe pages. A crucial step in staying gluten free will be keeping your pantry well stocked with gluten-free food. This will allow you to prepare any number of tasty meals at a moment's notice. All it takes is having the right ingredients and seasonings on hand.

In the previous chapters, we talked about some handy kitchen utensils that make producing gluten-free meals a breeze. That's the same with these foods. They allow you to whip up great meals without effort. Some of these foods you'll need to eat and replace weekly; others keep for months. The more you experiment with the recipes, meals, and snacks that work for you, the better sense you'll have of what you need to shop for.

One thing you'll notice is the proliferation of gluten-free foods available at the neighborhood grocery store (not to mention restaurants and bakeries). But if you're looking for more guidance on locating gluten-free-friendly brands, these online resources may come in handy:

- **AMERICANCELIAC.ORG** (American Celiac Disease Alliance)
- **CELIACCENTRAL.ORG** (National Foundation for Celiac Awareness)
- **CELIAC.ORG** (Celiac Disease Foundation)
- **CSACELIACS.ORG** (Celiac Support Association)
- **GLUTENFREELIVING.COM** (*Gluten-Free Living* magazine)
- **GLUTEN.NET** (Gluten Intolerance Group of North America)
- **LIVINGWITHOUT.COM** (*Living Without* magazine)

Gluten-Free Pantry and Shopping List

BAKING ESSENTIALS

__ Cornstarch	__ Cornmeal	__ Baking powder
__ Baking soda	__ Vanilla extract	__ Xanthan gum or guar gum
__ Sugar	__ Gluten-free all-	__ Gluten-free baking mixes
__ Gluten-free	purpose flour	(such as breads, cakes,
pancake/waffle mix	(a blend of flours)	cookies, and brownies)

DAIRY

__ Milk	__ Plain yogurt	__ Cheese (not processed)
__ Buttermilk	__ Greek yogurt	__ Eggs and egg substitute
__ Plain cream cheese	__ Dairy-free milks	

GRAINS, CEREALS, PASTA, AND RICE

__ Amaranth
__ Flaxseed
__ White, wild, and
   brown rice (plain)
__ Gluten-free
   corn tortillas
__ Gluten-free waffles

__ Buckwheat
__ Millet
__ Gluten-free cold
   and hot cereals
__ Gluten-free bread,
   sandwich buns, rolls

__ Cornmeal or plain grits
__ Quinoa
__ Corn, bean, potato, quinoa,
   rice, and soy pastas
__ Gluten-free cereal bars

MEAT, FISH, POULTRY, AND MEATLESS PROTEIN SOURCES

__ Fresh or frozen
   (plain and not
   injected with broth)
__ Gluten-free deli meats

__ Plain nuts
__ Peanut and
   other nut butters

__ Dried beans and lentils
__ Canned beans and lentils
__ Tofu (plain)

CONDIMENTS, SAUCES, AND SPICES

__ Ketchup
__ Mayonnaise
__ Mustard (plain)
__ Relish
__ Honey and molasses
__ Hummus

__ Guacamole
__ Jams and jellies
__ Gelatin
__ Vinegar
__ Lower-sodium
   gluten-free soy sauce

__ Assorted spices (see page 44)
__ Tomato sauce
__ Gluten-free stock and broth
__ Gluten-free sauce packets
__ Gluten-free seasoning
   packets

FRUITS AND VEGETABLES

__ Fresh or frozen

__ Dried

__ Canned (in juice or water)

FATS AND OILS

__ Butter or
   buttery spread

__ Vegetable, olive,
   and canola oils

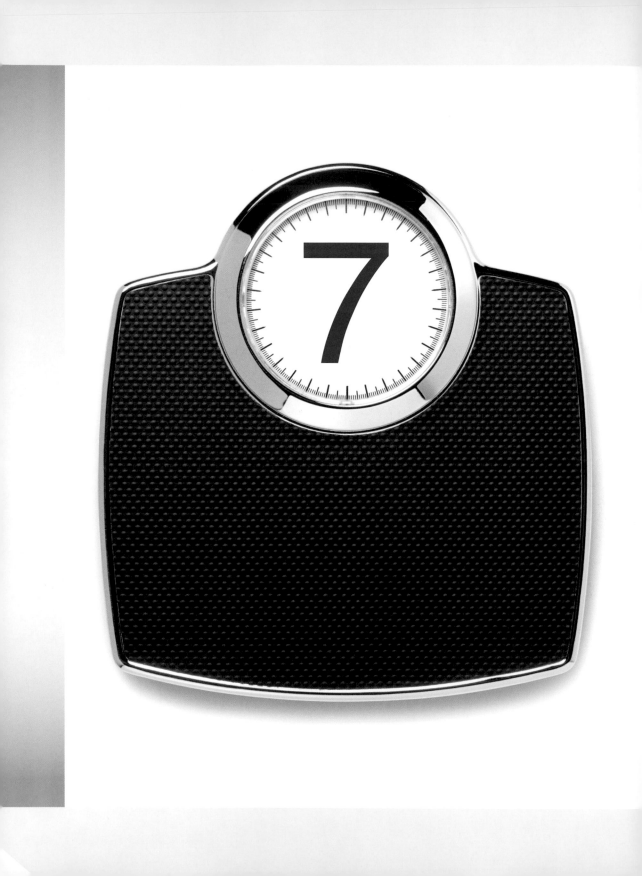

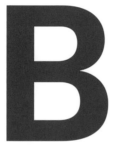**REAKFAST IS AN IMPORTANT MEAL—AND ONE OF THE TASTIEST.** In this chapter, you'll find an assortment of recipes that will hopefully offer you something new to add to your morning rotation, whether you're looking for quick breakfasts for busy weekdays or dishes for more relaxed weekend meals.

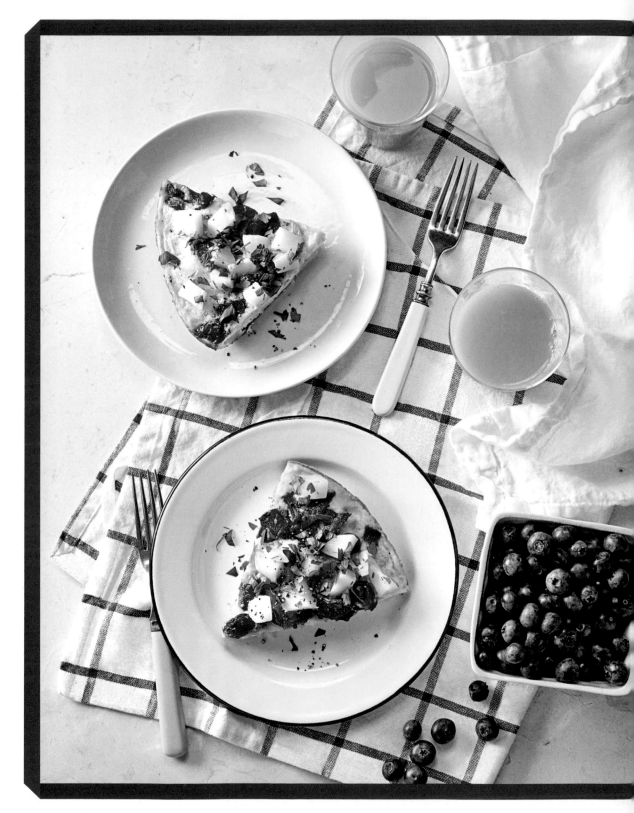

Peppery Potato Omelet

1½   pounds Yukon gold potatoes, peeled and cut into ½-inch pieces
1   large red bell pepper
1   tablespoon extra-virgin olive oil
2½   cups thinly vertically sliced onion
3   large eggs, lightly beaten
3   large egg whites, lightly beaten
1   teaspoon kosher salt, divided
¼   teaspoon freshly ground black pepper
1   tablespoon chopped fresh parsley

1. Preheat broiler.

2. Place potatoes in a saucepan; cover with water. Bring to a boil. Reduce heat; simmer 8 minutes or until tender. Drain well.

3. Cut bell pepper in half lengthwise; discard seeds and membranes. Place bell pepper halves, skin sides up, on a foil-lined baking sheet; flatten with hand. Broil 8 minutes or until blackened. Place pepper halves in a paper bag; fold to close tightly. Let stand 10 minutes. Peel and chop.

4. Reduce oven temperature to 350°.

5. Heat a large nonstick ovenproof skillet over medium-high heat. Add oil. Add onion; sauté 5 minutes. Combine eggs, egg whites, and ½ teaspoon salt in a large bowl; stir with a whisk. Pour egg mixture over onions; top with potatoes. Sprinkle potatoes with bell pepper, ½ teaspoon salt, and black pepper. Cook 2 minutes, shaking pan. Place pan in oven; bake at 350° for 8 minutes or until eggs are set. Sprinkle with parsley.

YIELD | SERVES 8 (SERVING SIZE: 1 WEDGE)

CALORIES 149; FAT 3.8g (sat 0.9g, mono 2g, poly 0.6g); PROTEIN 6g; CARB 23g; FIBER 3g; CHOL 70mg; IRON 1mg; SODIUM 295mg; CALC 32mg

Mushroom Frittata

2	ounces finely grated fresh pecorino Romano cheese (about ½ cup)
¼	teaspoon freshly ground black pepper
8	large eggs
½	teaspoon salt, divided
1	tablespoon extra-virgin olive oil, divided
1	(8-ounce) package sliced mushrooms
¾	cup chopped green onions
⅓	cup chopped fresh basil
2	cups baby arugula
2	teaspoons lemon juice

1. Preheat oven to 350°.

2. Combine first 3 ingredients; add ¼ teaspoon salt, stirring with a whisk. Heat a 10-inch ovenproof skillet over medium-high heat. Add 2 teaspoons oil; swirl to coat. Add mushrooms and ¼ teaspoon salt; sauté 6 minutes or until mushrooms brown and most of liquid evaporates. Stir in onions; sauté 2 minutes. Reduce heat to medium. Add egg mixture and basil to pan, stirring gently to distribute vegetable mixture; cook 5 minutes or until eggs are partially set. Place pan in oven. Bake at 350° for 7 minutes or until eggs are cooked through and top is lightly browned. Remove pan from oven; let stand 5 minutes. Run a spatula around edge and under frittata to loosen from pan; slide frittata onto a plate or cutting board.

3. Combine 1 teaspoon oil, arugula, and lemon juice. Cut frittata into 6 wedges; top with arugula mixture.

YIELD | SERVES 6 (SERVING SIZE: 1 FRITTATA WEDGE AND ABOUT ⅓ CUP ARUGULA MIXTURE)

CALORIES 145; FAT 8.7g (sat 2.5g, mono 4.2g, poly 1.3g); PROTEIN 10g; CARB 4g; FIBER 0g; CHOL 243mg; IRON 2mg; SODIUM 352mg; CALC 87mg

Zucchini and Red Pepper Frittata

1   large red bell pepper
1   tablespoon olive oil
1   large zucchini, thinly sliced (about 2 cups)
4   ounces white cheddar cheese, shredded (about 1 cup)
¾   cup 2% reduced-fat milk or dairy-free alternative
¼   teaspoon salt
¼   teaspoon freshly ground black pepper
4   large eggs, lightly beaten

1. Preheat broiler.
2. Cut bell pepper in half lengthwise; discard seeds and membranes. Place bell pepper halves, skin sides up, on a foil-lined baking sheet; flatten with hand. Broil 8 minutes or until blackened. Place pepper halves in a paper bag; fold to close tightly. Let stand 10 minutes. Peel and slice.
3. Reduce oven temperature to 350°.
4. Heat a 9-inch nonstick ovenproof skillet over medium-high heat. Add oil to pan; swirl to coat. Add zucchini; cook 6 minutes. Stir in bell pepper; reduce heat to medium. Combine cheese and next 4 ingredients (through eggs) in a large bowl. Add to zucchini mixture; cook 2 minutes or until edges are set. Bake at 350° for 16 minutes or until center is set.
5. Let stand 15 minutes. Cut into 6 wedges.

YIELD | SERVES 6 (SERVING SIZE: 1 WEDGE)

CALORIES 175; FAT 12.4g (sat 5.2g, mono 3g, poly 1g); PROTEIN 11g; CARB 6g; FIBER 1g; CHOL 147mg; IRON 1mg; SODIUM 294mg; CALC 201mg

INGREDIENT TIP
Frittata fillings
These easy egg dishes are open to endless interpretations. Feel free to substitute your favorite vegetables and cheeses.

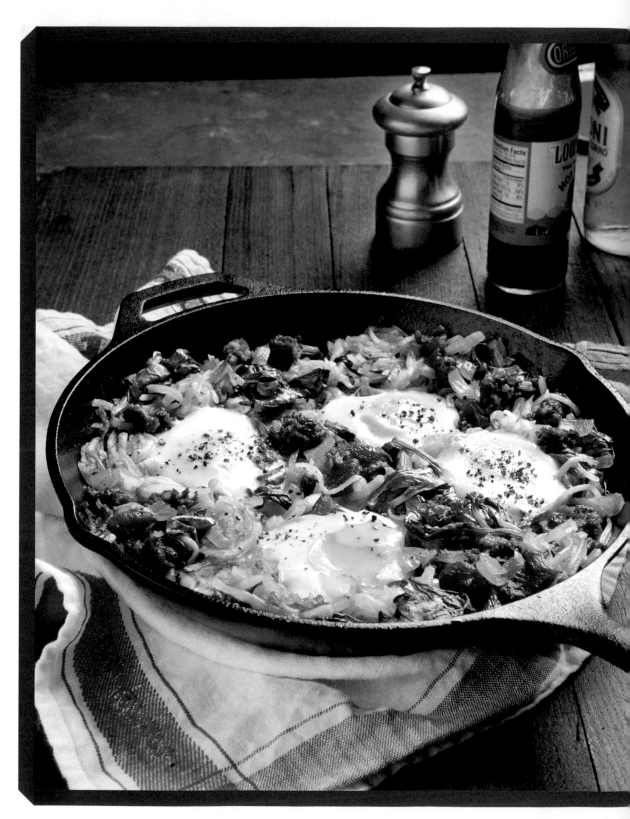

Mexican Chorizo Hash

This breakfast-for-dinner skillet gets heat from spicy Mexican chorizo. Don't stir the potatoes too much as they cook, so they crisp in the pan.

2	ounces Mexican chorizo
1	cup chopped onion
¼	cup coarsely chopped bottled roasted red bell peppers
½	teaspoon kosher salt
½	teaspoon freshly ground black pepper
1	(6-ounce) package baby spinach
2	teaspoons olive oil
2½	cups refrigerated gluten-free shredded hash brown potatoes
4	large eggs

1. Heat a large skillet over medium-high heat. Add chorizo to pan; cook 3 minutes or until browned, stirring to crumble. Add onion, bell pepper, salt, and black pepper; cook 3 minutes, stirring occasionally. Add spinach; stir until spinach wilts. Remove sausage mixture from pan. Add oil to pan; swirl to coat. Add potatoes; cook 8 minutes or until bottom is crisp. Stir in sausage mixture. Make 4 egg-sized spaces in pan with a spoon. Crack 1 egg into each space. Cover and cook 4 minutes or until egg yolks are slightly set.

YIELD | SERVES 4 (SERVING SIZE: ABOUT 1 CUP POTATO MIXTURE AND 1 EGG)

CALORIES 279; FAT 11.1g (sat 3.9g, mono 3.5g, poly 1.2g); PROTEIN 13g; CARB 33g; FIBER 5g; CHOL 206mg; IRON 2mg; SODIUM 616mg; CALC 68mg

Cheesy Hash Brown Casserole

1   cup gluten-free unsalted chicken stock
2   cups chopped onion, divided
2   (8-ounce) packages presliced white mushrooms, divided
6   garlic cloves
½   cup light sour cream
4   ounces reduced-fat sharp cheddar cheese, shredded and divided (about 1 cup)
1   teaspoon freshly ground black pepper
½   teaspoon kosher salt
3   center-cut bacon slices
1   (30-ounce) package frozen gluten-free shredded hash brown potatoes, thawed
1   tablespoon olive oil, divided
2   large eggs, lightly beaten
2   ounces 40%-less-fat original kettle-style potato chips, crushed
3   tablespoons chopped fresh flat-leaf parsley

1. Preheat oven to 400°.

2. Combine stock, 1 cup onion, half of mushrooms, and garlic in a saucepan; bring to a boil. Cover, reduce heat, and simmer 10 minutes or until mushrooms are tender. Place mixture in a blender. Remove center piece of lid (to allow steam to escape); secure blender lid on blender. Place a towel over opening in lid (to avoid splatters); blend until smooth. Stir in sour cream, 2 ounces cheese, pepper, and salt; blend until smooth.

3. Cook bacon in a large cast-iron skillet over medium heat until crisp. Remove bacon from pan; crumble. Add half of potatoes to drippings in pan; cover and cook 4 minutes on each side or until browned. Remove potatoes from pan. Repeat procedure with remaining potatoes and 2 teaspoons oil. Remove from pan.

4. Add 1 teaspoon oil to pan; swirl to coat. Add 1 cup onion and remaining mushrooms; cook 6 minutes or until tender. Return potatoes to pan; add eggs, stirring well to combine. Pour sour cream mixture over potato mixture. Sprinkle with bacon, 2 ounces cheese, chips, and parsley. Bake at 400° for 10 minutes or until cheese melts. Turn broiler on (do not remove pan from oven); broil 1½ minutes or until lightly browned.

YIELD | SERVES 8 (SERVING SIZE: 1 WEDGE)

CALORIES 273; FAT 9.7g (sat 4g, mono 2.9g, poly 0.7g); PROTEIN 13g; CARB 34g; FIBER 3g; CHOL 63mg; IRON 1mg; SODIUM 379mg; CALC 178mg

Sunflower Granola

1	cup certified gluten-free old-fashioned rolled oats	½	teaspoon ground cinnamon
¼	cup raw sunflower seed kernels	¼	teaspoon salt
¼	cup shredded sweetened coconut	2	tablespoons butter, melted
¼	cup chopped walnuts	2	tablespoons honey
¼	cup flaxseed meal	½	teaspoon vanilla extract

1. Place oven rack on middle shelf, about 10 inches below broiler. Preheat broiler.

2. Combine first 7 ingredients on a baking sheet; toss well. Broil 3 minutes or until lightly toasted, stirring every 1 minute. Combine butter, honey, and vanilla in a small bowl. Drizzle butter mixture over oat mixture; toss to coat. Broil 2 minutes or until well toasted, stirring after 1 minute. Remove granola from oven; cool on pan 8 minutes, stirring occasionally.

YIELD | SERVES 8 (SERVING SIZE: ¼ CUP)

CALORIES 159; FAT 10.4g (sat 3.3g, mono 2.4g, poly 4g); PROTEIN 4g; CARB 15g; FIBER 3g; CHOL 8mg; IRON 1mg; SODIUM 107mg; CALC 15mg

Pumpkinseed-Almond Granola

½	cup certified gluten-free old-fashioned rolled oats	5	teaspoons brown sugar
¼	cup unsalted pumpkinseed kernels, roasted	1½	tablespoons canola oil
1	ounce lightly salted smoked almonds, chopped	1	teaspoon grated orange rind
		1	tablespoon fresh orange juice
		¼	teaspoon vanilla extract
		⅛	teaspoon salt

1. Preheat oven to 325°.

2. Combine all ingredients in a medium bowl, stirring well with a spatula. Spread mixture on a parchment paper–lined baking sheet. Bake at 325° for 26 minutes. Cool completely.

YIELD | SERVES 4

CALORIES 195; FAT 13.4g (sat 1.4g, mono 6.9g, poly 4g); PROTEIN 5g; CARB 16g; FIBER 2g; CHOL 0mg; IRON 1mg; SODIUM 107mg; CALC 24mg

Vanilla Amaranth with Peach Compote

2   teaspoons butter
1   cup uncooked amaranth
2   cups 1% low-fat milk or dairy-free alternative
Dash of salt
½   vanilla bean (split lengthwise)
¾   pound sliced peaches (fresh or frozen)
¼   cup water
2   tablespoons sugar
⅛   teaspoon ground cinnamon
Dash of ground ginger

1. Melt butter in a medium saucepan over medium heat. Add amaranth; cook 2 minutes. Stir in milk, dash of salt, and vanilla bean; bring to a boil. Cover, reduce heat, and simmer 20 minutes or until liquid is absorbed. Discard vanilla bean.
2. Combine peaches, ¼ cup water, sugar, cinnamon, and dash of ground ginger in a saucepan over medium-high heat; bring to a boil. Simmer 12 minutes or until peaches are tender and thick. Serve peaches over amaranth.

YIELD | SERVES 4 (SERVING SIZE: ½ CUP AMARANTH AND ⅓ CUP FRUIT)

CALORIES 310; FAT 6.7g (sat 2.7g, mono 1.7g, poly 1.5g); PROTEIN 11g; CARB 53g; FIBER 5g; CHOL 0mg; IRON 0mg; SODIUM 58mg; CALC 0mg

Savory Buckwheat with Tomato, Cheddar, and Bacon

This gluten-free, polenta-like cereal packs 41 grams of whole grains into one serving.

⅔ cup cooked cereal (such as Bob's Red Mill Creamy Buckwheat Hot Cereal)

1 center-cut bacon slice, cooked and crumbled

2 tablespoons reduced-fat shredded cheddar cheese

2 tablespoons chopped tomato

Slivered jalapeño pepper

1. Top cooked cereal with cooked and crumbled bacon, shredded cheddar cheese, chopped tomato, and slivered jalapeño pepper.

YIELD | SERVES 1

CALORIES 194; FAT 4g (sat 1.6g, mono 0.3g, poly 0.1g); PROTEIN 11g; CARB 31g; FIBER 3g; CHOL 10mg; IRON 1mg; SODIUM 223mg; CALC 101mg

Quinoa with Strawberries and Buttermilk

¾ cup cooked quinoa (such as Ancient Harvest Traditional Organic)

¼ cup low-fat buttermilk

½ cup sliced strawberries

2 tablespoons sliced almonds, toasted

1 teaspoon honey

1. Combine cooked quinoa and buttermilk in a microwave-safe bowl. Microwave at HIGH 45 seconds. Stir; let stand 1 minute. Top with sliced strawberries, almonds, and honey.

YIELD | SERVES 1

CALORIES 305; FAT 9.1g (sat 0.8g, mono 3.7g, poly 1.5g); PROTEIN 11g; CARB 47g; FIBER 7g; CHOL 2mg; IRON 3mg; SODIUM 75mg; CALC 139mg

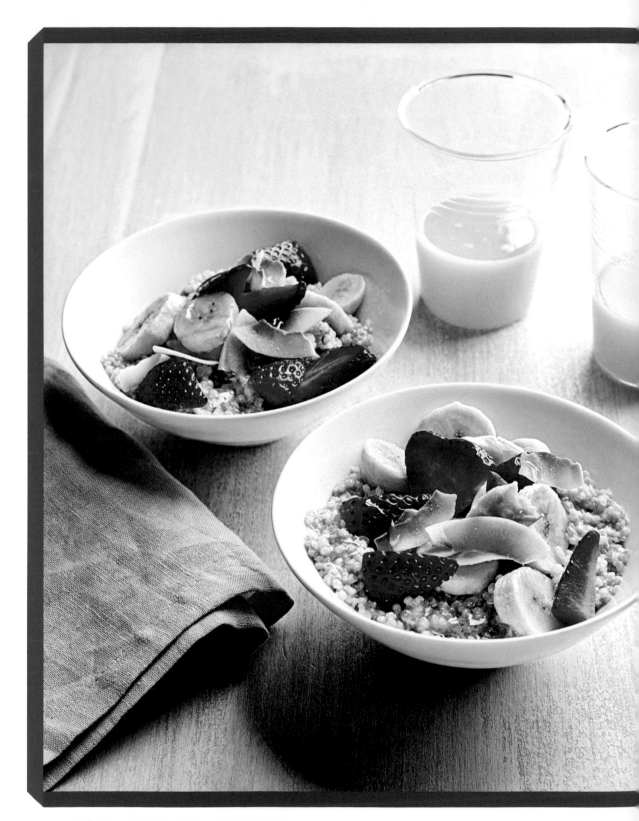

Breakfast Quinoa

Like most whole grains, quinoa is surprisingly filling, but if you need more for breakfast, serve with an egg on the side.

- ½   cup uncooked quinoa
- ¾   cup light coconut milk
- 2   tablespoons water
- 1   tablespoon brown sugar
- ⅛   teaspoon salt
- ¼   cup flaked unsweetened coconut
- 1   cup sliced strawberries
- 1   cup sliced banana

1. Preheat oven to 400°.
2. Place quinoa in a fine sieve, and place the sieve in a large bowl. Cover quinoa with water. Using your hands, rub grains together 30 seconds; rinse and drain quinoa. Repeat procedure twice. Drain well. Combine quinoa, coconut milk, 2 tablespoons water, brown sugar, and salt in a medium saucepan; bring to a boil. Reduce heat, and simmer 15 minutes or until liquid is absorbed, stirring occasionally. Stir mixture constantly during the last 2 minutes of cooking.
3. While quinoa cooks, spread flaked coconut in a single layer on a baking sheet. Bake at 400° for 5 minutes or until golden brown. Cool slightly.
4. Place about ½ cup quinoa mixture in each of 4 bowls. Top each serving with ¼ cup strawberry slices, ¼ cup banana slices, and 1 tablespoon toasted coconut. Serve warm.

YIELD | SERVES 4

CALORIES 178; FAT 5.5g (sat 3.8g, mono 0.4g, poly 0.8g); PROTEIN 4g; CARB 30g; FIBER 4g; CHOL 0mg; IRON 2mg; SODIUM 89mg; CALC 22mg

Oatmeal Pancakes

Now that potato starch and flours like tapioca flour are more widely available, it's easy to make your own gluten-free mix from scratch and have this mix on hand for whenever the urge for pancakes or waffles strikes.

Oatmeal Pancake and Waffle Mix:

4   ounces certified gluten-free oat flour (about 1 cup)
2.7   ounces potato starch (about ½ cup)
1.1   ounces tapioca flour (about ¼ cup)
2   tablespoons sugar
2   tablespoons baking powder
1   tablespoon flaxseed meal
2   teaspoons baking soda
⅛   teaspoon salt
½   cup certified gluten-free old-fashioned rolled oats

Remaining ingredients:

1½   cups low-fat buttermilk
¼   cup butter, melted
2   large egg whites, beaten

1. To prepare Oatmeal Pancake and Waffle Mix, weigh or lightly spoon oat flour, potato starch, and tapioca flour into dry measuring cups; level with a knife. Combine flours, potato starch, and next 5 ingredients (through salt) in a medium bowl, stirring well with a whisk. Add oats, stirring with a whisk.

2. Combine buttermilk, butter, and egg whites; add to mix, stirring until smooth. Pour ¼ cup batter per pancake onto a hot nonstick griddle or nonstick skillet. Cook 1 to 2 minutes or until tops are covered with bubbles and edges look cooked. Carefully turn pancakes over; cook 1 to 2 minutes or until bottoms are lightly browned.

YIELD | SERVES 7 (SERVING SIZE: 2 PANCAKES)

CALORIES 242; FAT 9.2g (sat 4.6g, mono 2.8g, poly 1.8g); PROTEIN 7g; CARB 33g; FIBER 3g; CHOL 20mg; IRON 1mg; SODIUM 355mg; CALC 143mg

Blueberry-Almond Oatmeal Pancakes

These blueberry pancakes get a double dose of almond flavor from the nuts and almond extract. Almond extract can be bitter when used in excess, so don't be tempted to add more—this amount is just right. If fresh blueberries are in season, feel free to substitute them for the frozen called for in the recipe.

2½	cups Oatmeal Pancake and Waffle Mix (page 80)
1½	cups low-fat buttermilk
¼	cup butter, melted
2	tablespoons maple syrup
¼	teaspoon almond extract
2	large egg whites, beaten
1	cup frozen small blueberries
1	tablespoon certified gluten-free oat flour
½	cup sliced almonds, toasted
1¼	cups maple syrup

1. Lightly spoon mix into dry measuring cups; level with a knife. Place mix in a large bowl. Combine buttermilk and next 4 ingredients (through egg whites), stirring with a whisk; add to mix, stirring until smooth. Let stand 10 minutes.

2. Combine blueberries and oat flour, tossing to coat. Fold blueberry mixture and almonds into batter.

3. Pour about ¼ cup batter per pancake onto a hot nonstick griddle or nonstick skillet. Cook 2 to 3 minutes or until tops are covered with bubbles and edges look cooked. Carefully turn pancakes over; cook 2 to 3 minutes or until bottoms are lightly browned. Serve with maple syrup.

YIELD | SERVES 10 (SERVING SIZE: 2 PANCAKES AND 2 TABLESPOONS SYRUP)

CALORIES 319; FAT 8.9g (sat 3.4g, mono 3.2g, poly 1.8g); PROTEIN 6g; CARB 56g; FIBER 3g; CHOL 14mg; IRON 1mg; SODIUM 254mg; CALC 157mg

Pecan-Oatmeal Waffles

Toasted pecans add a nutty sweetness to these oatmeal waffles flavored with cinnamon. Topped with sliced bananas and strawberries, with a swirl of maple syrup for added sweetness, they make a festive, pretty breakfast for your family or brunch for a crowd.

2½ cups Oatmeal Pancake and Waffle Mix (page 80)
¼ teaspoon ground cinnamon
1½ cups low-fat buttermilk
¼ cup butter, melted
2 tablespoons maple syrup
1 teaspoon vanilla extract
2 large egg whites, beaten
⅓ cup chopped pecans, toasted
Cooking spray
1 cup (⅛-inch-thick) slices banana
1 cup sliced strawberries
½ cup maple syrup

1. Lightly spoon mix into dry measuring cups; level with a knife. Combine mix and cinnamon in a large bowl, stirring with a whisk. Combine buttermilk and next 4 ingredients (through egg whites), stirring with a whisk; add to mix, stirring until smooth. Fold in pecans. Let stand 10 minutes.
2. Coat a round waffle iron with cooking spray; preheat.
3. Spoon about ½ cup batter per waffle onto hot waffle iron, spreading batter to edges. Cook 1½ minutes or until steaming stops; repeat procedure with remaining batter. Top waffles with banana and strawberry slices. Serve with syrup.

YIELD | SERVES 8 (SERVING SIZE: 1 WAFFLE, ABOUT ¼ CUP FRUIT, AND 1 TABLESPOON SYRUP)

CALORIES 336; FAT 11.7g (sat 4.4g, mono 4.2g, poly 2.1g); PROTEIN 6g; CARB 53g; FIBER 4g; CHOL 17mg; IRON 1mg; SODIUM 315mg; CALC 159mg

Mixed Berry Muffins

3.45 ounces brown rice flour (about ¾ cup)

2.6 ounces potato starch (about ½ cup)

1.8 ounces certified gluten-free oat flour (about ½ cup)

⅓   cup granulated sugar

¼   cup packed brown sugar

1½   teaspoons baking powder

1   teaspoon xanthan gum

½   teaspoon salt

½   cup 1% low-fat milk or dairy-free alternative

¼   cup butter, melted

2   large eggs

1½   cups mixed fresh berries (such as blueberries, raspberries, and blackberries)

     Cooking spray

1   tablespoon turbinado sugar or granulated sugar

1. Preheat oven to 350°.

2. Weigh or lightly spoon brown rice flour, potato starch, and oat flour into dry measuring cups; level with a knife. Combine brown rice flour, potato starch, oat flour, granulated sugar, and next 4 ingredients (through salt) in a medium bowl; stir with a whisk. Make a well in center of mixture. Combine milk, butter, and eggs, and stir with a whisk. Add to flour mixture, stirring just until moist. Fold in berries.

3. Place 12 paper muffin cup liners in muffin cups; coat liners with cooking spray. Spoon batter into prepared cups, and sprinkle with turbinado sugar. Bake at 350° for 25 minutes or until lightly browned and muffins spring back when lightly touched. Cool 10 minutes in pan on a wire rack; remove from pan.

Note: If you're planning to freeze all or some of the muffins, leave off the turbinado sugar.

YIELD | SERVES 12 (SERVING SIZE: 1 MUFFIN)

CALORIES 172; FAT 5.6g (sat 3g, mono 1.7g, poly 0.6g); PROTEIN 3g; CARB 28g; FIBER 2g; CHOL 42mg; IRON 1mg; SODIUM 206mg; CALC 70mg

INGREDIENT TIP

Oat flour If you can't find oat flour in your grocery store, make your own. Just place certified gluten-free oats in a food processor, and grind into a powdery consistency.

Cinnamon, Apple, and Oat Scones

4.2   ounces sweet white sorghum flour (about 1 cup)
1.3   ounces white rice flour (about ¼ cup)
1.2   ounces brown rice flour (about ¼ cup)
1.3   ounces potato starch (about ¼ cup)
1   cup certified gluten-free quick-cooking oats
¼   cup packed brown sugar
2   teaspoons baking powder
1   teaspoon xanthan gum
1   teaspoon baking soda
½   teaspoon salt
½   teaspoon ground cinnamon
¼   teaspoon ground nutmeg
5   tablespoons chilled unsalted butter, cut into small pieces
1   cup finely diced, peeled Granny Smith apple
¼   cup cinnamon-flavored baking chips
½   cup low-fat buttermilk
¼   cup applesauce
      White rice flour, for dusting
1   egg white, lightly beaten
2   teaspoons turbinado sugar or granulated sugar

1. Preheat oven to 400°.

2. Weigh or lightly spoon flours and potato starch into dry measuring cups; level with a knife. Combine flours, potato starch, oats, and next 7 ingredients (through nutmeg), stirring with a whisk; cut in butter with a pastry blender or 2 knives until mixture resembles coarse meal. Stir in apple and baking chips. Add buttermilk and applesauce; stir just until moist.

3. Turn dough out onto a surface lightly dusted with white rice flour. Pat dough into an 8-inch circle; cut into 14 wedges. Place wedges on a baking sheet lined with parchment paper. Brush egg white over surface of dough; sprinkle with turbinado sugar. Bake at 400° for 14 minutes or until golden brown. Serve warm.

Note: If you're planning to freeze all or some of the scones, leave off the turbinado sugar.

YIELD | SERVES 14 (SERVING SIZE: 1 SCONE)

CALORIES 169; FAT 6.1g (sat 3.3g, mono 1.3g, poly 0.3g); PROTEIN 3g; CARB 26g; FIBER 2g; CHOL 11mg; IRON 1mg; SODIUM 269mg; CALC 67mg

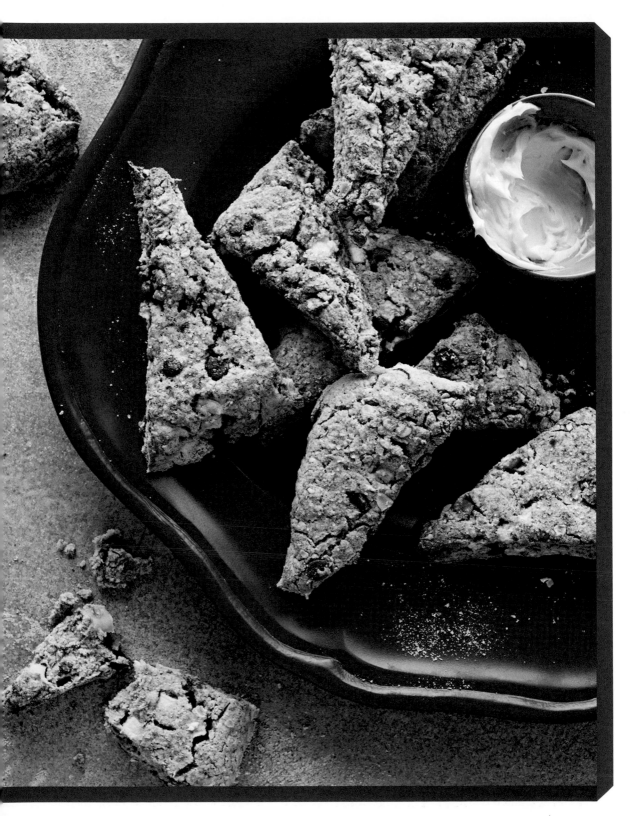

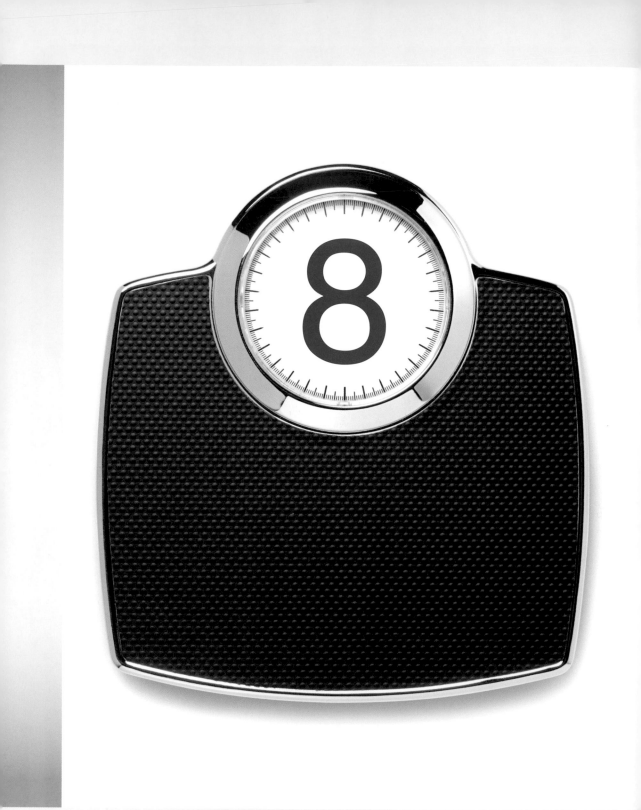

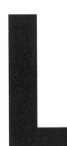

LUNCH IS OFTEN A MEAL GRABBED ON THE GO OR EATEN AT YOUR DESK. It might also consist of leftovers that you're not exactly looking forward to. The goal with this chapter is to offer you some fresh ideas to make your midday meal something a little more special.

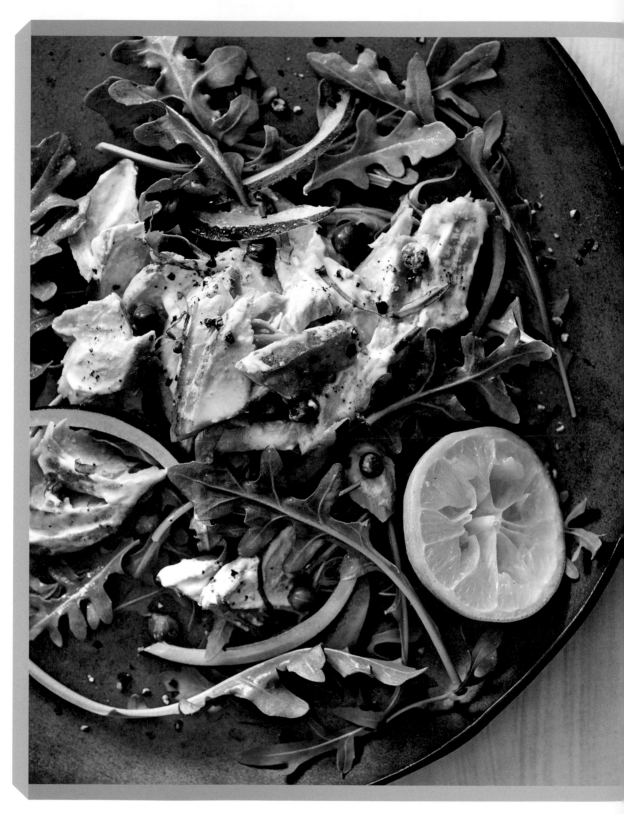

Salmon Salad on Arugula

One serving of this tasty fresh fish salad packs in a full day's worth of omega-3 fatty acids. Keep refrigerated in an airtight container up to two days.

4	(6-ounce) salmon fillets, skinned
¼	teaspoon kosher salt
¼	teaspoon black pepper
2	tablespoons olive oil, divided
2	tablespoons fresh lemon juice, divided
2	tablespoons plain fat-free Greek yogurt
2	tablespoons crème fraîche or sour cream
2	tablespoons thinly sliced fresh basil
4	teaspoons capers, rinsed, drained, and chopped
4	cups baby arugula leaves
1	cup very thinly vertically sliced red onion

1. Sprinkle salmon with salt and pepper. Heat a medium nonstick skillet over medium-high heat. Add 1 tablespoon oil to pan; swirl to coat. Add salmon; cook 6 minutes on each side or until fish flakes easily when tested with a fork or until desired degree of doneness. Cool to room temperature; flake with a fork.

2. Combine salmon, 1 tablespoon juice, yogurt, and next 3 ingredients (through capers) in a medium bowl. Refrigerate 30 minutes or up to 3 hours.

3. Combine 1 tablespoon oil, 1 tablespoon juice, arugula, and onion in a bowl. Toss gently to coat. Divide arugula mixture among 4 plates. Top with salmon mixture.

YIELD | SERVES 4 (SERVING SIZE: 1 CUP ARUGULA AND ⅔ CUP SALMON MIXTURE)

CALORIES 354; FAT 19.4g (sat 4.6g, mono 8.6g, poly 4g); PROTEIN 38g; CARB 5g; FIBER 1g; CHOL 97mg; IRON 1mg; SODIUM 297mg; CALC 65mg

Spicy Bean and Quinoa Salad with "Mole" Vinaigrette

To make this salad ahead, leave out the greens and keep the quinoa mixture covered in the refrigerator up to two days. Add the spinach just before serving.

1	teaspoon grated orange rind
2	tablespoons fresh orange juice
1½	tablespoons red wine vinegar
1	tablespoon adobo sauce from canned chipotle chiles in adobo sauce
¾	teaspoon unsweetened cocoa
½	teaspoon ground cumin
½	teaspoon ground cinnamon
2	tablespoons olive oil
3	cups cooked quinoa, at room temperature
½	cup unsalted pumpkinseed kernels, toasted
¼	cup chopped fresh cilantro
½	teaspoon kosher salt
2	green onions, thinly sliced
1	Fresno chile or jalapeño pepper, very thinly sliced
1	(15-ounce) can black beans, rinsed and drained
4	cups baby spinach leaves

1. Combine first 7 ingredients in a bowl; gradually add oil, stirring well with a whisk.

2. Combine quinoa and next 6 ingredients (through beans) in a large bowl. Add vinaigrette; toss to coat. Add spinach; toss to combine.

YIELD | SERVES 6 (SERVING SIZE: 1⅔ CUPS)

CALORIES 258; FAT 11.6g (sat 1.5g, mono 5.2g, poly 2.4g); PROTEIN 10g; CARB 31g; FIBER 7g; CHOL 0mg; IRON 4mg; SODIUM 377mg; CALC 55mg

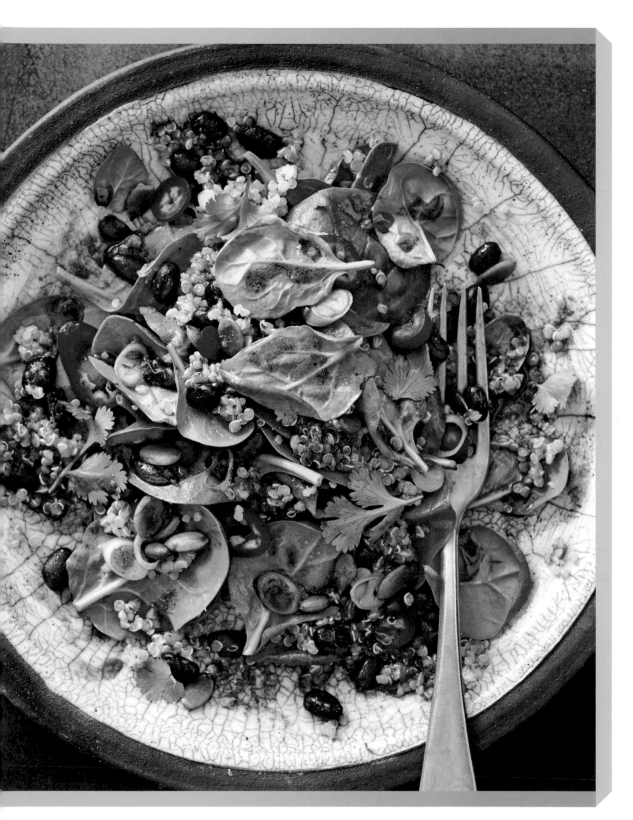

Warm Brown Rice and Chickpea Salad with Cherries and Goat Cheese

Fresh cherries add a meaty bite and tart-sweet flavor. If you can't find fresh cherries, add 2 tablespoons boiling water to ¼ cup unsweetened dried cherries. Let stand 10 minutes; drain and chop.

1   (8.8-ounce) pouch precooked brown rice (such as Uncle Ben's)
¼   cup chopped green onions
¼   cup chopped fresh basil
3   tablespoons extra-virgin olive oil
2   tablespoons white balsamic vinegar
½   teaspoon salt
¼   teaspoon freshly ground black pepper
32 cherries, pitted and quartered
1   (15-ounce) can unsalted chickpeas, rinsed and drained
2   ounces crumbled goat cheese (about ½ cup)

1. Heat rice according to package directions. Place rice in a medium bowl. Stir in onions and next 7 ingredients (through chickpeas). Sprinkle with goat cheese.

YIELD | SERVES 4 (SERVING SIZE: 1 CUP)

CALORIES 359; FAT 16.8g (sat 4.6g, mono 8.4g, poly 1.2g); PROTEIN 10g; CARB 43g; FIBER 5g; CHOL 11mg; IRON 2mg; SODIUM 389mg; CALC 100mg

Roasted Carrot, Chicken, and Grape Quinoa Bowl

2 cups (¾-inch) diagonally cut carrot
2 teaspoons olive oil
½ teaspoon kosher salt, divided
Cooking spray
5 tablespoons plain 2% reduced-fat Greek yogurt
3 tablespoons fresh lemon juice
2 tablespoons water
1½ tablespoons honey
¾ teaspoon ground cumin
½ teaspoon freshly ground black pepper
1½ cups cooked quinoa
1½ cups shredded skinless, boneless rotisserie chicken breast
1½ cups seedless red grapes, halved
½ cup thinly sliced green onions
½ cup fresh flat-leaf parsley leaves
½ cup sliced almonds, toasted
4 cups mixed salad greens

1. Preheat oven to 450°.
2. Combine carrot, oil, and ¼ teaspoon salt on a jelly-roll pan coated with cooking spray; toss to coat. Bake at 450° for 15 minutes or until tender.
3. Combine ¼ teaspoon salt, yogurt, and next 5 ingredients (through pepper) in a large bowl, stirring with a whisk. Add carrot, quinoa, and next 5 ingredients (through almonds); toss. Place 1 cup salad greens in each of 4 shallow bowls; top each serving with about 1½ cups quinoa mixture.

YIELD | SERVES 4

CALORIES 371; FAT 12.3g (sat 1.6g, mono 6.2g, poly 2g); PROTEIN 25g; CARB 44g; FIBER 7g; CHOL 51mg; IRON 3mg; SODIUM 502mg; CALC 142mg

Blueberry Chicken Salad

12 ounces shredded skinless, boneless rotisserie chicken (about 3 cups)	2½ tablespoons fresh lemon juice, divided
½ cup thinly vertically sliced red onion	1 tablespoon honey
⅓ cup diced celery	2 cups fresh blueberries
¼ cup torn fresh basil	1 (5-ounce) package baby arugula
½ teaspoon kosher salt, divided	2 teaspoons extra-virgin olive oil
½ cup plain 2% reduced-fat Greek yogurt	¼ teaspoon freshly ground black pepper

1. Combine first 4 ingredients in a medium bowl; sprinkle with ¼ teaspoon salt. Combine yogurt, 1 tablespoon lemon juice, and honey in a small bowl, stirring with a whisk. Add yogurt mixture to chicken mixture; toss to coat. Gently stir in blueberries. Place arugula, 1½ table-spoons lemon juice, oil, ¼ teaspoon salt, and pepper in a bowl; toss to coat. Divide arugula mixture among 6 plates; top each serving with about ¾ cup chicken mixture.

YIELD | SERVES 6

CALORIES 188; FAT 8.5g (sat 2.1g, mono 3.9g, poly 1.3g); PROTEIN 16g; CARB 13g; FIBER 2g; CHOL 75mg; IRON 1mg; SODIUM 369mg; CALC 69mg

Tuna-Pecan Salad Sandwiches

⅓ cup chopped celery	1 (12-ounce) can albacore tuna in water, drained
⅓ cup diced Gala apple (about 1 small)	
⅓ cup fat-free mayonnaise	4 curly leaf lettuce leaves
¼ cup chopped pecans, toasted	4 gluten-free English muffins, split and toasted
¼ teaspoon salt	
¼ teaspoon freshly ground black pepper	

1. Combine first 7 ingredients in a small bowl. Place a lettuce leaf on half of each English muffin. Top with tuna salad. Top with remaining English muffin halves.

YIELD | SERVES 4 (SERVING SIZE: 1 SANDWICH)

CALORIES 302; FAT 9.5 (sat 1g, mono 3.7g, poly 3.6g); PROTEIN 18g; CARB 47g; FIBER 4g; CHOL 18mg; IRON 4mg; SODIUM 752mg; CALC 19mg

Spicy Steak Lettuce Wraps

These wraps give traditional lettuce wraps a kick in the taste buds with the addition of zesty-spiced steak.

- 1   (12-ounce) sirloin steak, trimmed
- 2   tablespoons dark brown sugar
- 3   tablespoons rice vinegar
- 3   tablespoons gluten-free lower-sodium soy sauce
- 2   tablespoons grated shallots
- 2   tablespoons sambal oelek (ground fresh chile paste)
- 1   tablespoon grated peeled fresh ginger
- 2   teaspoons sesame oil
- Cooking spray
- 12 large Boston lettuce leaves (about 2 heads)
- 1   cup matchstick-cut English cucumber
- 1   cup thinly sliced red onion
- 1   cup matchstick-cut carrots
- ½   cup fresh cilantro leaves

1. Place steak in freezer 15 minutes. Remove from freezer; cut across grain into ⅛-inch-thick slices. Combine sugar and next 6 ingredients (through oil) in a large zip-top plastic bag; seal bag, and shake. Remove 3 tablespoons marinade, and set aside. Add steak to marinade in bag; seal and shake. Marinate in refrigerator 1 hour. Remove steak from bag; discard marinade. Heat a large skillet over medium-high heat. Coat pan with cooking spray. Add steak to pan, and cook 1 minute on each side.

2. Divide steak among lettuce leaves. Top each leaf with 4 teaspoons cucumber, 4 teaspoons onion, 4 teaspoons carrots, and 2 teaspoons cilantro; drizzle with reserved 3 tablespoons marinade.

YIELD | SERVES 4 (SERVING SIZE: 3 LETTUCE WRAPS)

CALORIES 268; FAT 13.5g (sat 4.7g, mono 5.6g, poly 1.5g); PROTEIN 19g; CARB 18g; FIBER 2g; CHOL 64mg; IRON 2mg; SODIUM 363mg; CALC 57mg

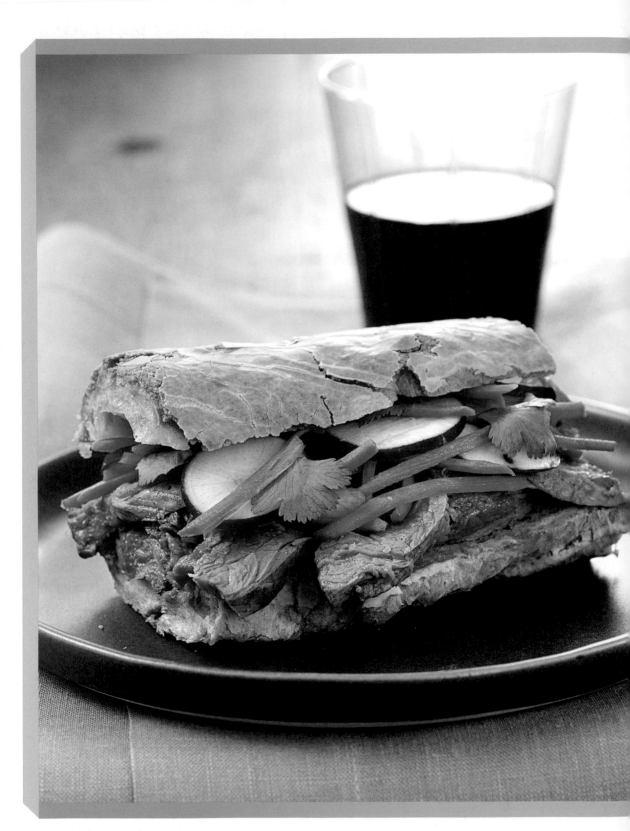

Banh Mi–Style Roast Beef Sandwiches

⅛   teaspoon freshly ground black pepper

1   (¾-pound) flank steak, trimmed

2   tablespoons rice vinegar

1   tablespoon fish sauce (such as Thai Kitchen)

1   tablespoon lower-sodium gluten-free soy sauce

1½   teaspoons sugar

1   jalapeño pepper, thinly sliced

1   cup matchstick-cut carrots

½   cup thinly sliced radishes

1   (7.5-ounce) gluten-free baguette or rolls, halved lengthwise and toasted

½   cup fresh cilantro leaves

1. Heat a large cast-iron skillet over medium-high heat. Sprinkle pepper over steak. Add steak to pan; cook 5 minutes on each side or until desired degree of doneness. Remove steak from pan; let stand 5 minutes. Cut steak diagonally across grain into thin slices.

2. While steak cooks, combine vinegar and next 4 ingredients (through jalapeño pepper) in a medium bowl. Combine carrots and radishes in a medium bowl; add 1 tablespoon vinegar mixture, tossing to coat. Let vegetable mixture stand 5 minutes. Add steak to remaining 5 tablespoons vinegar mixture; toss well to coat.

3. Arrange steak on bottom half of bread; top with vegetable mixture and cilantro. Top with top half of bread; cut into 4 equal pieces.

YIELD | SERVES 4 (SERVING SIZE: 1 SANDWICH)

CALORIES 355; FAT 12.8g (sat 2.9g, mono 4.8g, poly 2.5g); PROTEIN 28g; CARB 31g; FIBER 1g; CHOL 98mg; IRON 3mg; SODIUM 834mg; CALC 102mg

Pork Wraps with Fresh Tomatillo Salsa

2   large tomatillos
½   cup chopped cucumber
¼   cup chopped fresh cilantro
2   tablespoons fresh lime juice
½   teaspoon salt, divided
1   garlic clove, peeled
Cooking spray
1   pound boneless pork cutlets, cut into thin strips
1   teaspoon ground cumin
2   medium poblano chiles, stemmed, seeded, and cut into thin strips
1   medium onion, vertically sliced
4   (8-inch) gluten-free tortillas
½   cup light sour cream

INGREDIENT TIP

Warming tortillas

Since gluten-free tortillas are stored in the refrigerator, they'll need to be warmed to prevent breaking. You can steam them by placing each tortilla on a splatter guard set over a pan of simmering water. Cover with a lid, and heat about 5 to 10 seconds or until they're soft and pliable. Or you can warm them in the microwave (see page 103 for instructions).

1. Discard husks and stems from tomatillos. Place tomatillos, cucumber, cilantro, lime juice, ¼ teaspoon salt, and garlic in a blender. Process until finely chopped, and set aside.

2. Heat a large nonstick skillet over medium-high heat. Coat pan with cooking spray. Sprinkle pork with cumin. Add pork to pan; cook 3 minutes or until no longer pink in center, stirring occasionally. Remove from pan; keep warm.

3. Recoat pan with cooking spray; add chiles and onion. Coat vegetables with cooking spray; cook 4 minutes or until onion begins to brown, stirring frequently.

4. While vegetables cook, warm tortillas.

5. Return pork to pan; add ¼ teaspoon salt, and cook 30 seconds or until pork mixture is thoroughly heated, stirring constantly.

6. Divide pork mixture among tortillas. Top each with about ⅓ cup salsa; roll up. Serve with sour cream.

YIELD | SERVES 4 (SERVING SIZE: 1 WRAP AND 2 TABLESPOONS SOUR CREAM)

CALORIES 350; FAT 10.1g (sat 3.2g, mono 2.9g, poly 2.4g); PROTEIN 29g; CARB 36g; FIBER 6g; CHOL 85mg; IRON 3mg; SODIUM 468mg; CALC 57mg

Spicy Chicken Sandwiches

¼   cup reduced-fat mayonnaise
2   tablespoons chopped fresh cilantro
1   teaspoon fresh lime juice
1   garlic clove, minced
2   egg whites, lightly beaten
3   tablespoons hot pepper sauce (such as Tabasco)
1   teaspoon dried oregano
½   teaspoon salt
2   (6-ounce) skinless, boneless chicken breast halves
4½ ounces gluten-free tortilla chips (about 6 cups)
2   tablespoons olive oil
4   (1.5-ounce) gluten-free sandwich rolls
12 (⅛-inch-thick) slices red onion
4   lettuce leaves

1. Combine first 4 ingredients; refrigerate until ready to prepare sandwiches.

2. Combine egg whites and next 3 ingredients (through salt) in a large zip-top plastic bag. Cut chicken breast halves in half horizontally to form 4 cutlets. Add chicken to bag; seal. Marinate in refrigerator at least 2 hours or up to 8 hours, turning bag occasionally.

3. Place tortilla chips in a food processor; process 1 minute or until ground. Place ground chips in a shallow dish.

4. Working with 1 cutlet at a time, remove chicken from bag, allowing excess marinade to drip off. Coat chicken completely in chips. Set aside. Repeat procedure with remaining chicken and chips.

5. Heat a large nonstick skillet over medium heat. Add oil to pan, swirling to coat. Add chicken to pan; cook 3 minutes on each side or until browned and done. Spread mayonnaise mixture evenly over cut sides of rolls. Layer bottom half of each roll with 3 onion slices, 1 lettuce leaf, and 1 chicken cutlet; top with top halves of rolls.

YIELD | SERVES 4 (SERVING SIZE: 1 SANDWICH)

CALORIES 416; FAT 10.8g (sat 2g, mono 3.9g, poly 3.4g); PROTEIN 29g; CARB 56g; FIBER 8g; CHOL 54mg; IRON 1mg; SODIUM 802mg; CALC 408mg

Spicy-Sweet Chicken Lettuce Cups

A quick vinegar soak keeps the chicken moist and intensely flavorful in this dish.

- 2   cups cider vinegar
- 1   cup water
- ½   cup sugar
- 2   tablespoons sliced serrano chile
- ¾   teaspoon kosher salt
- 1   small garlic clove, crushed
- 1   cup matchstick-cut carrots
- 1½ cups shredded skinless, boneless rotisserie chicken breast
- 1½ cups shredded skinless, boneless rotisserie chicken thigh or drumstick
- 12 butter lettuce leaves
- 24 English cucumber slices
- 6   tablespoons dry-roasted peanuts, chopped
- ¼   cup torn fresh mint

1. Combine first 6 ingredients in a medium saucepan. Bring mixture to a boil; cook 20 minutes. Remove from heat. Stir in carrots; let stand 10 minutes to soften. Add chicken to carrot mixture; let stand 5 minutes. Drain and discard liquid.

2. Place about ¼ cup chicken mixture in each lettuce leaf, and top each lettuce leaf with 2 cucumber slices, 1½ teaspoons peanuts, and 1 teaspoon mint.

YIELD | SERVES 6 (SERVING SIZE: 2 LETTUCE CUPS)

CALORIES 147; FAT 7g (sat 1.4g, mono 3.2g, poly 1.6g); PROTEIN 18g; CARB 5g; FIBER 1g; CHOL 58mg; IRON 1mg; SODIUM 265mg; CALC 25mg

INGREDIENT TIP

Dark and light meat

A mix of chicken breast and thigh or drumstick gives these lettuce cups more richness, but feel free to use all white meat, if you prefer.

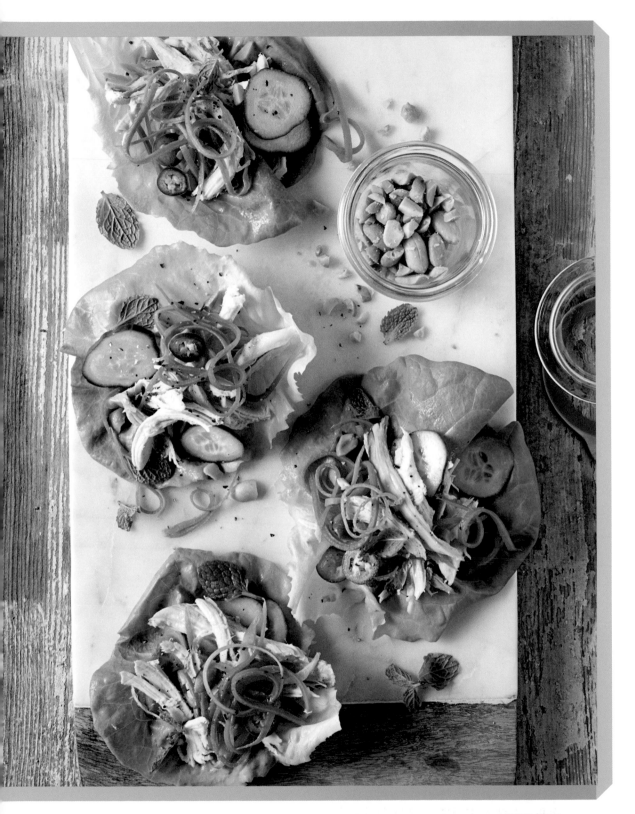

Chicken-Olive Quesadillas

3   ounces part-skim mozzarella cheese, shredded (about ¾ cup)
½   cup chopped cooked chicken breast
3   tablespoons sliced ripe olives
¼   teaspoon chili powder
¼   teaspoon ground cumin
1   (4-ounce) can chopped green chiles, drained
Butter-flavored cooking spray
4   (6-inch) corn tortillas
Fresh salsa (optional)
Reduced-fat sour cream (optional)

1. Combine first 6 ingredients in a medium bowl.

2. Heat a large nonstick skillet over medium-high heat. Coat pan with cooking spray. Add 1 tortilla to pan. Spread about ½ cup chicken mixture on left half of tortilla; fold right side of tortilla over filling, pressing gently with a spatula. Place an additional tortilla in pan, overlapping first quesadilla. Spread about ½ cup chicken mixture on right half of tortilla; fold left side of tortilla over filling, pressing with spatula. (Folded sides of tortillas should meet in center of pan.) Cook 1 minute.

3. Coat quesadillas with cooking spray; turn quesadillas over, keeping folded sides together in center of pan. Cook 1 to 2 minutes or until golden and cheese melts. Remove from pan; cover and keep warm. Repeat procedure with cooking spray and remaining tortillas and filling. Serve immediately with salsa and sour cream, if desired.

YIELD | SERVES 4 (SERVING SIZE: 1 QUESADILLA)

CALORIES 178; FAT 6.3g (sat 1.4g, mono 2.6g, poly 1.8g); PROTEIN 12g; CARB 16g; FIBER 1g; CHOL 15mg; IRON 0mg; SODIUM 312mg; CALC 9mg

Portobello and Black Bean Quesadillas

4   (8-inch) gluten-free tortillas
Butter-flavored cooking spray
2   (4½-inch) portobello mushroom caps, chopped
1   cup canned unsalted black beans, rinsed and drained
2   tablespoons light balsamic vinaigrette
1   (2-ounce) jar diced pimiento, drained
4   ounces preshredded reduced-fat 4-cheese Mexican blend cheese
    (about 1 cup)
¼   cup thinly sliced green onions
Fresh salsa (optional)
Reduced-fat sour cream (optional)

1. Stack tortillas; microwave at HIGH 1 minute. Leave in microwave to keep warm while preparing filling.
2. Heat a large nonstick skillet over medium-high heat. Coat pan with cooking spray. Add mushrooms; sauté 2 minutes or until tender. Add beans, vinaigrette, and pimiento; cook 1 to 2 minutes or until liquid evaporates, stirring constantly. Mash bean mixture slightly with a potato masher.
3. Spoon about ⅓ cup bean mixture onto each tortilla. Sprinkle with cheese and onions. Fold tortillas in half.
4. Wipe pan with paper towels; heat over medium heat. Coat pan with cooking spray. Place 2 quesadillas in pan; cook 2 to 3 minutes on each side or until golden and cheese melts. Repeat procedure with remaining 2 quesadillas. Cut each quesadilla into 3 wedges. Serve immediately with salsa and sour cream, if desired.

YIELD | SERVES 4 (SERVING SIZE: 1 QUESADILLA)

CALORIES 289; FAT 9.3g (sat 3.4g, mono 2.2g, poly 1.5g); PROTEIN 14g; CARB 38g; FIBER 6g; CHOL 18mg; IRON 2mg; SODIUM 512mg; CALC 364mg

Broccoli-Cheese Soup

Traditional broccoli-cheese soup has nearly 400 calories and more than 18 grams of saturated fat per serving. Ours has fewer than half the calories and one-fourth of the saturated fat.

3	cups unsalted gluten-free chicken stock
1¾	cups broccoli florets, coarsely chopped (about 8 ounces)
1	cup diced yellow onion
½	cup chopped carrot
⅜	teaspoon salt
¼	teaspoon freshly ground black pepper
2	garlic cloves, minced
4	ounces reduced-fat extra-sharp cheddar cheese, shredded and divided (about 1 cup)
¾	cup half-and-half
¼	cup fresh flat-leaf parsley leaves

1. Combine first 7 ingredients in a large saucepan; bring to a boil. Reduce heat, and simmer 10 minutes or until broccoli is tender. Pour soup into a blender. Remove center piece of blender lid (to allow steam to escape); secure lid on blender. Place a clean towel over opening in blender lid (to avoid splatters). Blend until smooth. Return soup to pan. Stir in 2 ounces cheese and half-and-half. Top with remaining cheese and parsley.

YIELD | SERVES 4 (SERVING SIZE: ABOUT 1 CUP SOUP AND 2 TABLESPOONS CHEESE)

CALORIES 160; FAT 7.4g (sat 4.5g, mono 2.1g, poly 0.3g); PROTEIN 14g; CARB 11g; FIBER 2g; CHOL 23mg; IRON 1mg; SODIUM 532mg; CALC 213mg

Black Bean Soup

1   cup dried black beans
2½   tablespoons extra-virgin olive oil, divided
¾   cup chopped onion
7   garlic cloves, minced and divided
2½   cups gluten-free, fat-free, lower-sodium chicken broth
2   cups water
¼   cup unsalted tomato paste
1   teaspoon dried oregano
¾   teaspoon salt
¾   teaspoon ground cumin
¼   teaspoon ground red pepper
1   (4-ounce) can chopped green chiles
1   cup fresh cilantro leaves
½   jalapeño pepper, seeded
¼   cup Mexican crema
3   hard-cooked large eggs, peeled and finely chopped

1. Sort and wash beans, and place in a large Dutch oven. Cover with water; cover and let stand 8 hours. Drain beans.

2. Heat 1½ teaspoons oil in a Dutch oven over medium heat. Add onion; cook 4 minutes, stirring often. Add 5 garlic cloves; cook 1 minute. Increase heat to medium-high. Add beans, broth, and next 7 ingredients (through chiles); bring to a boil. Cover, reduce heat, and simmer 1 hour or until beans are tender. Let stand 10 minutes.

3. Place half of bean mixture in a blender. Remove center piece of blender lid (to allow steam to escape); secure blender lid on blender. Place a clean towel over opening in blender lid (to avoid splatters). Blend until smooth. Pour into a large bowl. Repeat procedure with remaining mixture. Return soup to pan; cook 5 minutes, stirring often.

4. Finely chop 1 cup cilantro and jalapeño. Combine 2 tablespoons oil, 2 garlic cloves, cilantro, jalapeño, and crema. Ladle 1¼ cups soup into each of 4 bowls; top each with 2 tablespoons crema mixture. Sprinkle soup with eggs.

YIELD | SERVES 4

CALORIES 369; FAT 18.4g (sat 5.8g, mono 7.8g, poly 1.8g); PROTEIN 18g; CARB 35g; FIBER 12g; CHOL 173mg; IRON 5mg; SODIUM 829mg; CALC 114mg

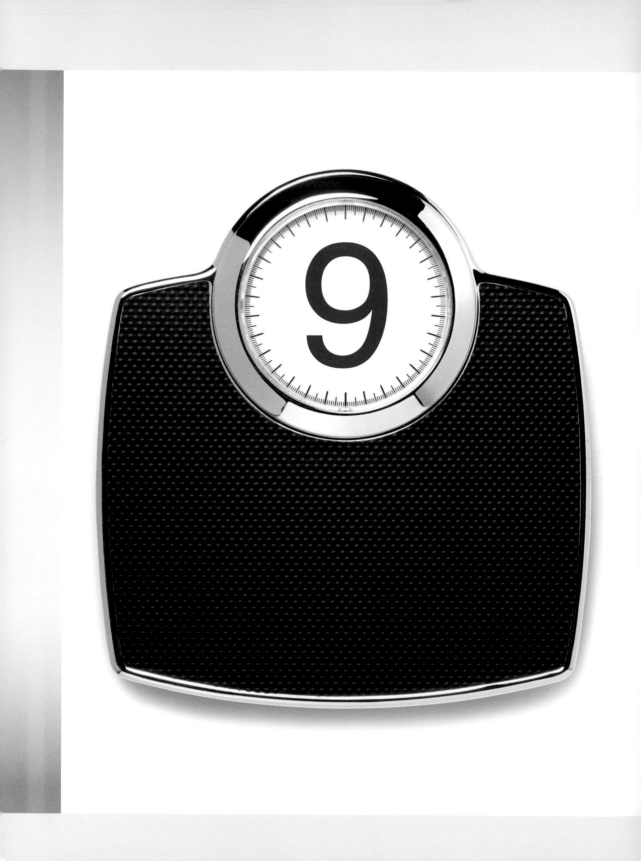

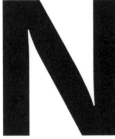

DINNER

NO MATTER WHAT DIET YOU ARE ON, KEEPING DINNER FRESH CAN BE CHALLENGING. This chapter offers an array of healthy meals that will provide something tasty for everyone around your dinner table—even if they aren't eating gluten free.

Salsa Flounder

Serve this dish with rice or corn tortillas.

- 1 tablespoon olive oil
- 4 (6-ounce) flounder fillets
- ½ teaspoon salt-free Cajun/Creole seasoning
- ½ cup thinly sliced shallots (about 2 shallots)
- 1 tablespoon butter, melted
- 2 garlic cloves, thinly sliced
- ¾ cup fresh salsa
- ¼ teaspoon freshly ground black pepper
- 1 tablespoon coarsely chopped cilantro
- 4 lime wedges

1. Place oven rack in middle of oven. Preheat broiler.

2. Drizzle oil in a roasting pan. Pat fish dry with paper towels; arrange fish in pan. Sprinkle fish with Cajun seasoning. Sprinkle shallots, butter, and garlic around pan. Pour salsa into pan around fish. Broil 10 minutes or until fish flakes easily when tested with a fork or until desired degree of doneness, basting frequently. Arrange fish on a platter; sprinkle with pepper. Stir cilantro into pan sauce; drizzle sauce over fish. Serve with lime wedges.

YIELD | SERVES 4 (SERVING SIZE: 1 FILLET, ABOUT 2 TABLESPOONS SAUCE, AND 1 LIME WEDGE)

CALORIES 189; FAT 9.1g (sat 2.9g, mono 4g, poly 1g); PROTEIN 19g; CARB 6g; FIBER 1g; CHOL 73mg; IRON 1mg; SODIUM 567mg; CALC 41mg

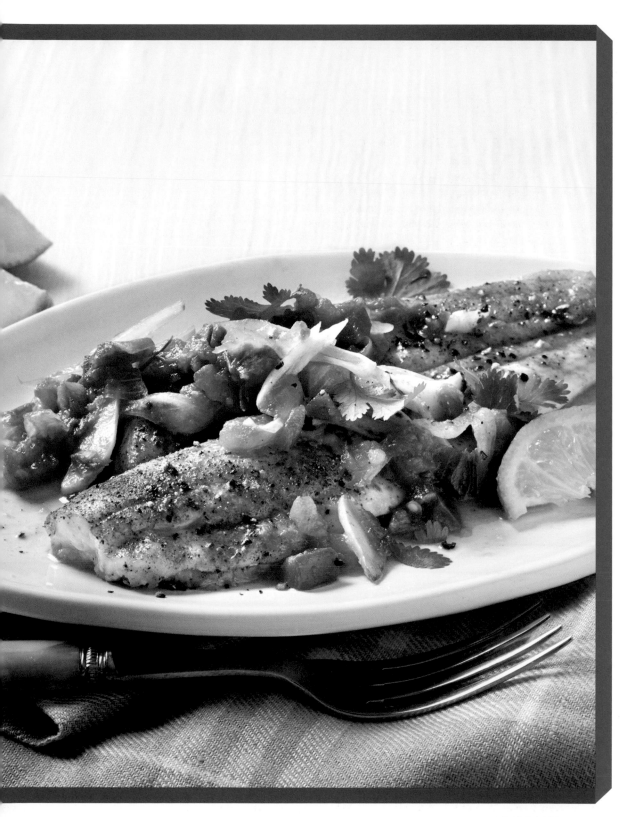

Cedar Plank Salmon with Tomato Salsa

1 (18-inch) cedar plank
1 poblano chile, seeded and halved
1 jalapeño pepper, seeded and halved
1 small red onion, cut into ½-inch-thick slices
Cooking spray
2 cups chopped seeded heirloom tomato
3 tablespoons chopped fresh cilantro
½ teaspoon kosher salt, divided
½ teaspoon freshly ground black pepper, divided
1 diced peeled avocado
1 lime, divided
4 (6-ounce) skinless salmon fillets

1. Soak plank in water 25 minutes.

2. Preheat grill to medium-high heat.

3. Place poblano, jalapeño, and onion on grill rack coated with cooking spray; grill 10 minutes, turning occasionally. Remove from grill; cool. Coarsely chop poblano and onion; finely chop jalapeño. Combine peppers, onion, tomato, cilantro, ¼ teaspoon salt, ¼ teaspoon pepper, avocado, and juice from half of lime.

4. Sprinkle fish with ¼ teaspoon salt and ¼ teaspoon black pepper. Place plank on grill rack; grill 3 minutes or until lightly charred. Turn plank over; place fish on charred side. Cover; grill 8 minutes or until desired degree of doneness. Cut remaining lime half into 4 wedges. Top each fillet with ½ cup tomato salsa. Serve with lime wedges.

YIELD | SERVES 4

CALORIES 386; FAT 20.7g (sat 4.2g, mono 10.6g, poly 4.2g); PROTEIN 38g; CARB 12g; FIBER 6g; CHOL 87mg; IRON 1mg; SODIUM 330mg; CALC 48mg

Saffron Rice with Tilapia and Shrimp

8   ounces unpeeled large shrimp
3⅓   cups gluten-free unsalted chicken stock
⅔   cup water
⅛   teaspoon saffron threads, crushed
1   cup chopped ripe tomato
1   cup chopped onion
1⅛   teaspoons salt, divided
½   teaspoon sugar
4   garlic cloves
3   tablespoons olive oil
1¼   cups uncooked short-grain rice
12   ounces tilapia, cut into 1-inch pieces
½   cup frozen green peas
¼   cup chopped fresh flat-leaf parsley
6   lemon wedges

1. Preheat oven to 450°.

2. Peel shrimp, reserving shells; set shrimp aside. Combine shrimp shells, chicken stock, ⅔ cup water, and saffron in a saucepan. Bring to a boil; reduce heat, and keep warm.

3. Combine tomato, onion, ½ teaspoon salt, sugar, and garlic in a food processor; process until smooth.

4. Heat a large ovenproof skillet over medium-high heat. Add oil to pan; swirl to coat. Add tomato mixture to pan; cook 6 minutes or until liquid almost evaporates, stirring occasionally. Add uncooked rice to pan; cook 3 minutes, stirring frequently. Drain stock mixture over a bowl; discard solids. Add stock mixture to pan; bring to a boil. Cook over medium heat 12 minutes or until rice is tender and liquid is absorbed (do not stir). Top with reserved shrimp, tilapia, and peas. Sprinkle with ⅝ teaspoon salt. Cover and bake at 450° for 15 minutes or until fish flakes easily when tested with a fork or until desired degree of doneness. Sprinkle with parsley; serve with lemon wedges.

YIELD | SERVES 6 (SERVING SIZE: ABOUT 1½ CUPS RICE MIXTURE AND 1 LEMON WEDGE)

CALORIES 338; FAT 8.8g (sat 1.5g, mono 5.4g, poly 1.4g); PROTEIN 24g; CARB 41g; FIBER 3g; CHOL 76mg; IRON 3mg; SODIUM 600mg; CALC 60mg

INGREDIENT TIP

Shrimp shells

This paella-inspired dish starts by infusing purchased chicken stock with shrimpy goodness. It's an easy step that makes full use of shrimp shells that would have otherwise been discarded.

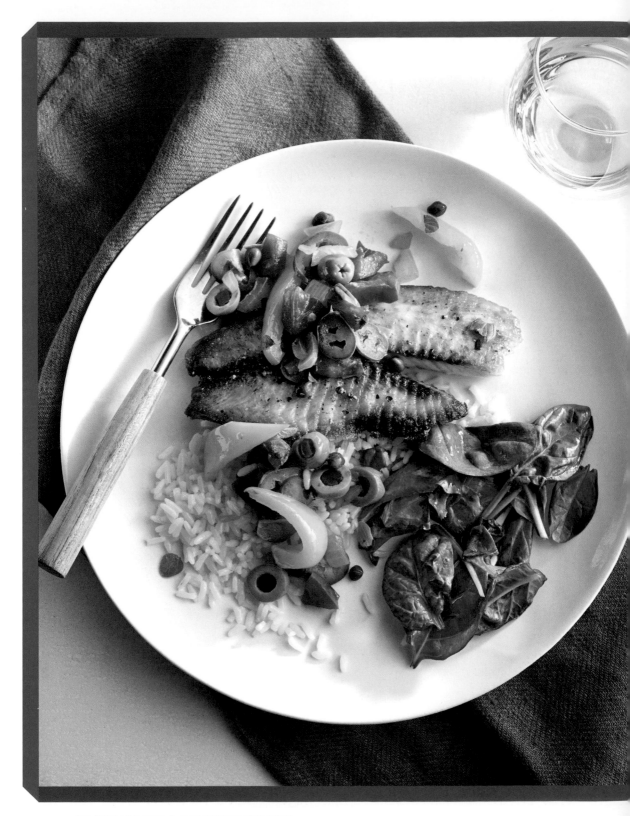

Tilapia Veracruz

Spanish and Mexican flavors combine in this quick fish dish.
Serve with steamed rice and sautéed spinach.

4	**(4-ounce) tilapia fillets**
½	**teaspoon freshly ground black pepper**
¼	**teaspoon salt**
1	**tablespoon extra-virgin olive oil**
1½	**cups chopped onion**
1	**tablespoon chopped fresh oregano**
4	**garlic cloves, sliced**
1	**yellow bell pepper, thinly sliced**
2	**cups chopped tomato**
2	**ounces pimiento-stuffed green olives (about 20), halved**
1	**tablespoon capers, rinsed and drained**
1	**jalapeño pepper, thinly sliced**

1. Sprinkle fish with pepper and salt. Heat a large nonstick skillet over medium-high heat. Add oil; swirl to coat. Add fish to pan; cook 3 minutes or until browned on one side. Remove fish from pan.

2. Add onion, oregano, garlic, and bell pepper to pan; sauté 4 minutes. Stir in tomato and remaining ingredients; bring to a simmer.

3. Arrange fish on top of tomato mixture, browned sides up. Cover, reduce heat to medium, and simmer 3 minutes or until fish flakes easily when tested with a fork or until desired degree of doneness.

YIELD | SERVES 4 (SERVING SIZE: 1 FILLET AND ½ CUP SAUCE)

CALORIES 211; FAT 7.2g (sat 1.2g, mono 4.1g, poly 1.4g); PROTEIN 25g; CARB 14g; FIBER 3g; CHOL 57mg; IRON 1mg; SODIUM 532mg; CALC 49mg

Sautéed Tilapia Tacos with Grilled Peppers and Onion

Slice the onion just before placing it on the grill. If given time to set, the onion rings will begin to separate and will not have good grill marks.

2	(½-inch-thick) slices white onion
1	(8-ounce) package mini sweet bell peppers
	Cooking spray
¾	teaspoon salt, divided
½	teaspoon freshly ground black pepper, divided
4	(5-ounce) tilapia fillets
8	(6-inch) corn tortillas
8	lime wedges (optional)

1. Preheat grill to high heat.

2. Arrange onion slices and bell peppers on a grill rack coated with cooking spray. Grill onions for 12 minutes, turning after 6 minutes. Grill bell peppers 12 minutes, turning occasionally. Remove onions and bell peppers from grill, and let stand for 5 minutes. Slice onion rings in half. Thinly slice bell peppers; discard stems and seeds. Combine onion, bell peppers, ¼ teaspoon salt, and ⅛ teaspoon black pepper in a small bowl.

3. Sprinkle fish evenly with ½ teaspoon salt and ⅜ teaspoon black pepper. Heat a large non-stick skillet over medium-high heat. Coat pan with cooking spray. Add fish to pan, and cook for 3 minutes on each side or until fish flakes easily when tested with a fork or until desired degree of doneness.

4. Warm tortillas according to package directions. Divide fish, onion mixture, and jalapeño slices evenly among tortillas. Serve with lime wedges, if desired.

YIELD | SERVES 4 (SERVING SIZE: 2 TACOS)

CALORIES 292; FAT 4.4g (sat 1.2g, mono 1.2g, poly 1.3g); PROTEIN 33g; CARB 32g; FIBER 5g; CHOL 71mg; IRON 2mg; SODIUM 526mg; CALC 120mg

Seared Scallops with Snap Peas and Pancetta

Sautéed snap peas, pancetta, and shallots make a speedy but sophisticated accompaniment to seared scallops.

- 3   teaspoons canola oil, divided
- 12   ounces sugar snap peas, trimmed and diagonally sliced
- ¼   teaspoon kosher salt, divided
- ¼   teaspoon black pepper, divided
- 1½   ounces diced pancetta (such as Boar's Head)
- 2   large shallots, sliced
- 1½   pounds large sea scallops
- 4   lemon wedges

1. Heat a large cast-iron skillet over medium-high heat. Add 1 teaspoon oil; swirl to coat. Add peas, ⅛ teaspoon salt, and ⅛ teaspoon pepper; sauté 2 minutes. Place peas in a bowl. Heat pan over medium heat. Add pancetta; cook 1 minute. Add shallots; cook 1 minute, stirring constantly. Add pancetta mixture to pea mixture.
2. Return pan to medium-high heat. Pat scallops dry with paper towels; sprinkle with ⅛ teaspoon salt and ⅛ teaspoon pepper. Add 1 teaspoon oil to pan; swirl to coat. Add half of scallops to pan; cook 2 minutes. Turn and cook 1 minute or until desired degree of doneness. Place cooked scallops on a plate. Repeat procedure with remaining 1 teaspoon oil and remaining scallops. Serve scallops with pea mixture and lemon wedges.

YIELD | SERVES 4 (SERVING SIZE: ABOUT 5 SCALLOPS AND ¾ CUP PEA MIXTURE)

CALORIES 237; FAT 7.9g (sat 2.2g, mono 2.3g, poly 1.3g); PROTEIN 25g; CARB 15g; FIBER 3g; CHOL 48mg; IRON 3mg; SODIUM 568mg; CALC 52mg

Asian Rice with Shrimp and Snow Peas

1	cup uncooked long-grain rice
1	cup water
1	cup gluten-free, fat-free, lower-sodium chicken broth
3	tablespoons gluten-free, lower-sodium soy sauce
3	tablespoons rice vinegar
1	tablespoon dark sesame oil
2	teaspoons minced fresh garlic
1	teaspoon hot sauce
2	cups snow peas, trimmed (about 6 ounces)
1½	pounds large peeled and deveined shrimp
½	cup diagonally cut green onions
4	teaspoons slivered almonds, toasted

1. Combine long-grain rice, 1 cup water, and broth in a medium saucepan; bring to a boil. Cover, reduce heat, and simmer 20 minutes or until liquid is absorbed.

2. Combine soy sauce, vinegar, sesame oil, garlic, and hot sauce in a large bowl; stir with a whisk. Set aside.

3. Cook snow peas and shrimp in boiling water 2 minutes or until shrimp are done. Drain. Add snow peas, shrimp, green onions, and rice to soy mixture; toss well to combine. Top with almonds. Serve immediately.

YIELD | SERVES 4 (SERVING SIZE: 2 CUPS SHRIMP MIXTURE AND 1 TEASPOON ALMONDS)

CALORIES 334; FAT 7.6g (sat 1.2g, mono 1.9g; poly 3.5g); PROTEIN 39g; CARB 25g; FIBER 2g; CHOL 259mg; IRON 6mg; SODIUM 776mg; CALC 129mg

Slow-Cooker Brisket

1	(4½-pound) flat-cut brisket roast, fat cap trimmed to ⅛-inch thickness
1¼	teaspoons kosher salt, divided
½	teaspoon freshly ground black pepper
1	tablespoon canola oil
1½	teaspoons garlic powder
1	teaspoon paprika
3	medium carrots, peeled and cut into thirds
3	celery stalks, cut into thirds
	Cooking spray
2	large onions, halved and vertically sliced
4	garlic cloves, chopped
1	cup gluten-free unsalted beef stock
2	tablespoons brown sugar
2	tablespoons cider vinegar
1	(15-ounce) can crushed tomatoes, undrained
5	thyme sprigs
2	bay leaves

1. Sprinkle brisket with 1 teaspoon salt and pepper. Heat a large skillet over medium-high heat. Add oil; swirl to coat. Add brisket; cook 5 minutes, turning to brown on all sides. Rub brisket with garlic powder and paprika. Arrange carrots and celery in a 6-quart electric slow cooker coated with cooking spray; top with brisket, fat cap side up.

2. Return pan to medium heat. Add onions to pan; cover and cook 10 minutes, stirring occasionally. Uncover. Stir in garlic; cook 5 minutes or until onions are tender and golden. Arrange onion mixture over brisket.

3. Combine ¼ teaspoon salt, stock, brown sugar, vinegar, and tomatoes in hot pan, stirring with a whisk to loosen browned bits. Pour tomato mixture around brisket. Place thyme and bay leaves in slow cooker, pressing into tomato mixture. Cover and cook on LOW 7 hours or until brisket is tender. Cool slightly in cooker, about 1 hour.

4. Place brisket on a cutting board. Trim fat cap; discard fat. Cut brisket across grain into thin slices. Pour sauce through a sieve over a bowl; discard carrots, celery, thyme, and bay leaves. Return onions to sauce. Serve brisket with sauce.

YIELD | SERVES 12 (SERVING SIZE: ABOUT 3 OUNCES BEEF AND ABOUT ⅔ CUP SAUCE)

CALORIES 307; FAT 15.1g (sat 5g, mono 7.1g, poly 0.8g); PROTEIN 33g; CARB 8g; FIBER 1g; CHOL 100mg; IRON 4mg; SODIUM 338mg; CALC 31mg

Cast-Iron Burgers

1	pound ground sirloin
¼	teaspoon kosher salt
1	tablespoon canola mayonnaise
1	tablespoon Dijon mustard
1	tablespoon prepared horseradish
2	teaspoons ketchup
2	applewood-smoked bacon slices, chopped
3	cups vertically sliced yellow onion
1	tablespoon finely chopped fresh chives
1	teaspoon gluten-free Worcestershire sauce
¼	teaspoon freshly ground black pepper
	Cooking spray
4	(2.8-ounce) gluten-free hamburger buns, toasted
4	green leaf lettuce leaves
4	(¼-inch-thick) slices tomato

1. Divide beef into 4 portions, lightly shaping each into a ½-inch-thick patty. Sprinkle with salt. Cover and refrigerate 30 minutes.

2. Combine mayonnaise and next 3 ingredients (through ketchup) in a small bowl. Set aside.

3. Cook bacon in a large nonstick skillet over medium-low heat until crisp. Remove bacon from pan. Add onion to drippings in pan; cook 15 minutes or until golden brown. Combine bacon, onion, chives, Worcestershire sauce, and pepper in a small bowl.

4. Heat a large cast-iron skillet over medium-high heat. Coat pan with cooking spray. Add patties; cook 2 minutes on each side or until desired degree of doneness. Spread 1½ teaspoons horseradish spread on cut side of each bun half. Top bottom half of each bun with 1 lettuce leaf, 1 tomato slice, 1 patty, ¼ cup relish, and top half of bun.

YIELD | SERVES 4 (SERVING SIZE: 1 BURGER)

CALORIES 420; FAT 16.6g (sat 5.9g, mono 5.9g, poly 1.5g); PROTEIN 30g; CARB 36g; FIBER 4g; CHOL 79mg; IRON 5mg; SODIUM 814mg; CALC 126mg

Roasted Pork Tenderloin Tacos

1   (1-pound) pork tenderloin, trimmed
½   teaspoon freshly ground black pepper
¼   teaspoon salt
1   tablespoon canola oil
2   tablespoons mojo marinade (such as Goya)
½   cup white wine vinegar
3   tablespoons water
1½ tablespoons sugar
1   cup thinly vertically sliced red onion
8   (6-inch) corn tortillas
1   jalapeño pepper, cut into 16 slices
1   ripe peeled avocado, cut into 16 wedges
¼   cup Mexican crema

1. Preheat oven to 425°.

2. Sprinkle pork with pepper and salt. Heat a large ovenproof skillet over medium-high heat. Add oil to pan; swirl to coat. Add pork; cook 5 minutes, turning to brown on all sides. Place pan in oven. Bake at 425° for 8 minutes or until a thermometer registers 145° (slightly pink); let stand 5 minutes. Cut crosswise into 16 slices. Combine pork and mojo marinade in a medium bowl; toss to coat pork.

3. Combine vinegar, 3 tablespoons water, and sugar in a small saucepan; bring to a boil. Remove from heat; add onion. Let stand 10 minutes; drain.

4. Working with 1 tortilla at a time, toast in a pan or over the flame of a gas burner until tender and blackened in spots. Arrange 2 pork slices in center of each tortilla; top with about 2 tablespoons onion, 2 jalapeño slices, 2 avocado wedges, and 1½ teaspoons crema.

YIELD | SERVES 4 (SERVING SIZE: 2 TACOS)

CALORIES 362; FAT 16.9g (sat 2.1g, mono 8g, poly 2.8g); PROTEIN 28g; CARB 27g; FIBER 6g; CHOL 82mg; IRON 2mg; SODIUM 423mg; CALC 55mg

INGREDIENT TIP

Mexican crema

Thick and slightly tangy Mexican crema adds a cooling finish to these tacos. If you can't find it at the grocery, substitute sour cream thinned with a little lime juice.

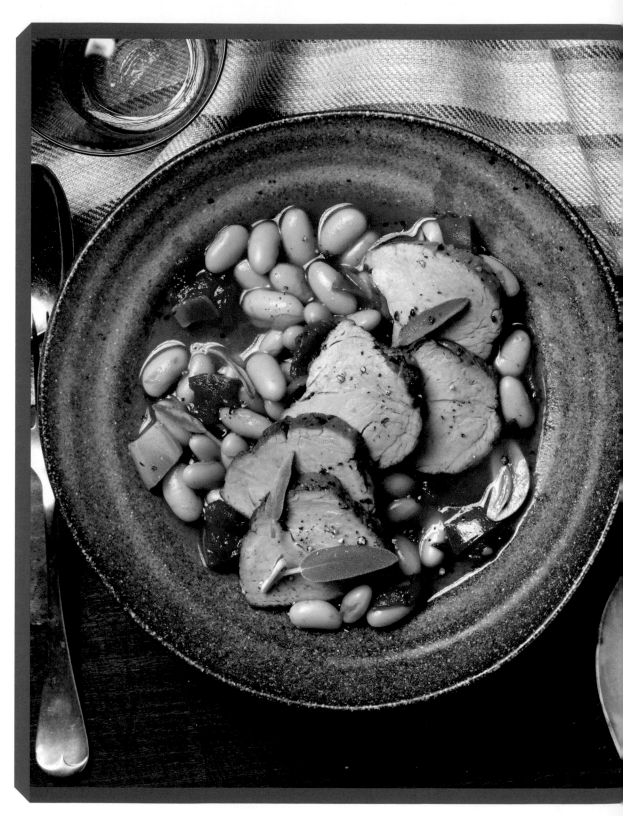

Pork Tenderloin and Cannellini Beans

1   teaspoon chopped fresh rosemary
¾   teaspoon kosher salt, divided
¾   teaspoon freshly ground black pepper, divided
½   teaspoon fennel seeds, lightly crushed
1   (1-pound) pork tenderloin, trimmed
1   tablespoon olive oil
½   cup chopped onion
4   large garlic cloves, thinly sliced
1   cup chopped tomato
1   teaspoon chopped fresh sage
1   cup gluten-free unsalted chicken stock
¼   teaspoon crushed red pepper
1   (15-ounce) can unsalted cannellini beans, rinsed and drained
2   tablespoons chopped fresh flat-leaf parsley

1. Preheat oven to 425°.

2. Combine rosemary, ½ teaspoon salt, ½ teaspoon black pepper, and fennel seeds in a small bowl. Rub spice mixture over pork.

3. Heat a large skillet over medium-high heat. Add oil; swirl to coat. Add pork; cook 9 minutes, browning on all sides. Remove pork from pan. Add onion and garlic; sauté 2 minutes. Add tomato and sage; cook 1 minute, scraping pan to loosen browned bits. Add ¼ teaspoon salt, ¼ teaspoon black pepper, stock, red pepper, and cannellini beans, and bring to a boil. Return pork to pan, and place pan in oven. Bake at 425° for 12 minutes or until a thermometer registers 140°.

4. Place pork on a cutting board; let stand 5 minutes. Heat pan over medium heat; cook bean mixture 2 minutes or until slightly thick. Sprinkle with parsley. Thinly slice pork; serve with bean mixture.

YIELD | SERVES 4 (SERVING SIZE: ABOUT 3 OUNCES PORK AND ½ CUP BEAN MIXTURE)

CALORIES 227; FAT 6.5g (sat 1.3g, mono 3.4g, poly 0.8g); PROTEIN 30g; CARB 13g; FIBER 3g; CHOL 74mg; IRON 2mg; SODIUM 475mg; CALC 51mg

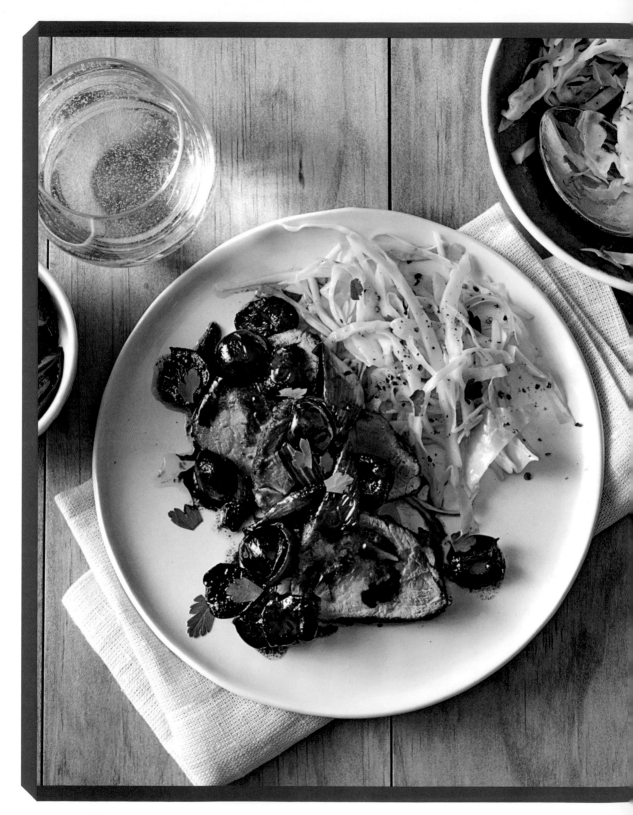

Pork Tenderloin with Roasted Cherries and Shallots

2   tablespoons canola oil, divided
¾   teaspoon kosher salt, divided
½   teaspoon freshly ground black pepper
½   teaspoon ground cumin
⅛   teaspoon ground cinnamon
1   (1-pound) pork tenderloin, trimmed
8   ounces fresh cherries, pitted and halved
3   large shallots, quartered
¼   cup gluten-free unsalted chicken stock
2   tablespoons balsamic vinegar
½   teaspoon brown sugar
1   tablespoon butter
¼   cup coarsely chopped fresh flat-leaf parsley

1. Preheat oven to 425°.

2. Heat a large ovenproof skillet over medium-high heat. Add 1 tablespoon oil; swirl to coat. Combine ½ teaspoon salt, pepper, cumin, and cinnamon. Rub pork with spice mixture. Add pork to pan; sauté 4 minutes. Turn pork over; place pan in oven and bake at 425° for 15 minutes or until a thermometer registers 140°. Remove pork from pan; place on a cutting board (do not wipe out pan). Let pork stand 10 minutes. Cut into thin slices.

3. Add 1 tablespoon oil to pan; swirl to coat. Add cherries and shallots; sprinkle with ¼ teaspoon salt. Place pan in oven; bake at 425° for 10 minutes (do not turn cherries). Carefully remove pan from oven; place over medium-high heat. Stir in stock, vinegar, and sugar; bring to a boil. Cook 4 minutes or until liquid is syrupy. Remove from heat; stir in butter. Serve cherry mixture with pork; sprinkle with parsley.

YIELD | SERVES 4 (SERVING SIZE: 3 OUNCES PORK AND ABOUT ⅔ CUP SAUCE)

CALORIES 270; FAT 12.5g (sat 3.2g, mono 6.1g, poly 2.5g); PROTEIN 25g; CARB 14g; FIBER 2g; CHOL 81mg; IRON 2mg; SODIUM 458mg; CALC 27mg

Citrus-Herb Chicken

Citrus zest perfumes the chicken while it marinates. A fresh salsa of citrus segments and herbs doubles down on fruit flavor.

2	large limes
1	large ruby red grapefruit
1	large tangerine
1	large navel orange
¼	cup extra-virgin olive oil, divided
1	tablespoon minced garlic
1	tablespoon minced serrano chile
1	(3½-pound) whole chicken
¾	teaspoon kosher salt, divided
⅜	teaspoon freshly ground black pepper, divided
1	cup vertically sliced red onion
¼	cup chopped fresh mint
2	tablespoons chopped fresh cilantro

1. Grate 1 teaspoon rind and squeeze 5 tablespoons juice from limes. Place rind and 4 tablespoons juice in a medium bowl; place 1 tablespoon juice in a separate medium bowl. Grate 1 teaspoon grapefruit rind; section grapefruit. Grate 1 teaspoon tangerine rind; section tangerine. Grate 1 teaspoon orange rind; section orange. Add citrus sections to 1 tablespoon lime juice in bowl; set aside. Add rinds to lime rind mixture. Add 2 tablespoons oil, garlic, and chile to rind mixture; stir with a whisk.

2. Place chicken, breast side down, on a cutting board. Using poultry shears, cut along both sides of backbone, and open chicken like a book. Turn chicken breast side up; using the heel of your hand, press firmly against the breastbone until it cracks. Lift wing tips up and over back; tuck under chicken. Discard backbone and skin. Place chicken on a rimmed baking sheet. Spread citrus rind mixture over chicken. Cover and refrigerate at least 4 hours.

3. Position oven rack in lower third of oven. Preheat broiler.

4. Sprinkle chicken with ½ teaspoon salt and ¼ teaspoon black pepper. Broil chicken, breast side down, 20 minutes. Turn chicken over; broil an additional 20 minutes or until done, turning pan occasionally. Let stand 10 minutes.

5. Combine reserved citrus section mixture, 2 tablespoons oil, ¼ teaspoon salt, ⅛ teaspoon pepper, red onion, mint, and cilantro; toss to combine.

YIELD | SERVES 4 (SERVING SIZE: ¼ OF CHICKEN AND ½ CUP SALSA)

CALORIES 369; FAT 17.6g (sat 2.9g, mono 11.1g, poly 2.4g); PROTEIN 31g; CARB 24g; FIBER 7g; CHOL 92mg; IRON 3mg; SODIUM 473mg; CALC 76mg

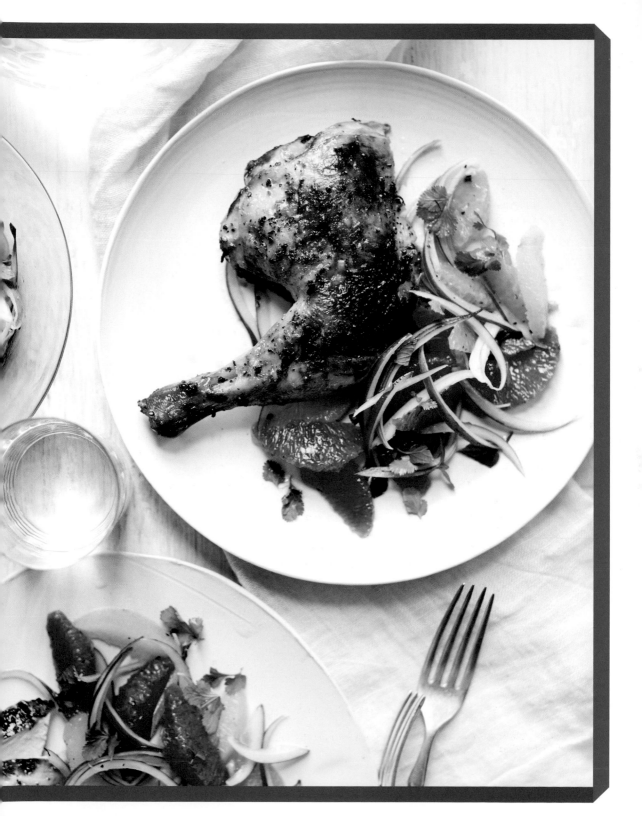

Chicken with Turnips and Pomegranate Sauce

3   cups gluten-free unsalted chicken stock, divided
1   cup uncooked wild rice
1   tablespoon chopped fresh thyme leaves
1¼   teaspoons black pepper, divided
¾   teaspoon kosher salt, divided
1   cup pomegranate juice
½   cup pomegranate arils
2   large turnips, peeled and cut into ¼-inch slices
2   tablespoons olive oil, divided
4   (6-ounce) skinless, boneless chicken breast halves

1. Preheat oven to 400°.
2. Combine 2 cups stock, rice, and thyme in a medium saucepan. Bring to a boil. Cover, reduce heat, and simmer 50 minutes. Drain. Stir in ½ teaspoon pepper and ¼ teaspoon salt.
3. Combine 1 cup stock and juice in a saucepan. Bring to a boil; reduce heat, and cook 20 minutes or until mixture is reduced to ⅓ cup. Remove from heat; stir in arils.
4. Combine turnips, ½ teaspoon pepper, ¼ teaspoon salt, and 1 tablespoon oil in a bowl; toss to coat. Arrange turnip mixture on a baking sheet. Bake at 400° for 20 minutes or until browned and tender, turning once.
5. Sprinkle ¼ teaspoon salt and ¼ teaspoon pepper over chicken. Heat a large ovenproof skillet over medium-high heat. Add 1 tablespoon oil to pan; swirl to coat. Add chicken; cook 4 minutes. Turn chicken, and place pan in oven. Bake at 400° for 8 minutes or until chicken is done.
6. Spoon about ½ cup rice onto each of 4 plates. Top with about ⅓ cup turnips and 1 chicken breast half. Drizzle each with about 4 teaspoons pomegranate sauce.

YIELD | SERVES 4

CALORIES 489; FAT 11.7g (sat 2g, mono 6.3g, poly 1.7g); PROTEIN 45g; CARB 51g; FIBER 4g; CHOL 109mg; IRON 2mg; SODIUM 678mg; CALC 68mg

Shredded Chicken Tacos with Tomatoes and Grilled Corn

2   ears shucked corn
1   (12-ounce) package baby heirloom tomatoes
½   teaspoon freshly ground black pepper
¼   teaspoon salt
8   (6-inch) corn tortillas
2   cups shredded skinless, boneless rotisserie chicken breast
1   peeled avocado, cut into 16 slices
8   lime wedges (optional)

1. Preheat broiler.
2. Place corn on a jelly-roll pan; broil 18 minutes or until charred on all sides, rotating every 6 minutes. Cut kernels from corn; place kernels in a medium bowl. Cut tomatoes into quarters. Add tomatoes to corn, and sprinkle corn mixture with black pepper and salt.
3. Heat tortillas according to package directions. Divide chicken evenly among tortillas; top each taco with ¼ cup corn mixture and 2 avocado slices. Serve with lime wedges, if desired.

YIELD | SERVES 4 (SERVING SIZE: 2 TACOS)

CALORIES 420; FAT 13.5g (sat 2.3g, mono 7.1g, poly 2.4g); PROTEIN 39g; CARB 41g; FIBER 8g; CHOL 101mg; IRON 2mg; SODIUM 554mg; CALC 123mg

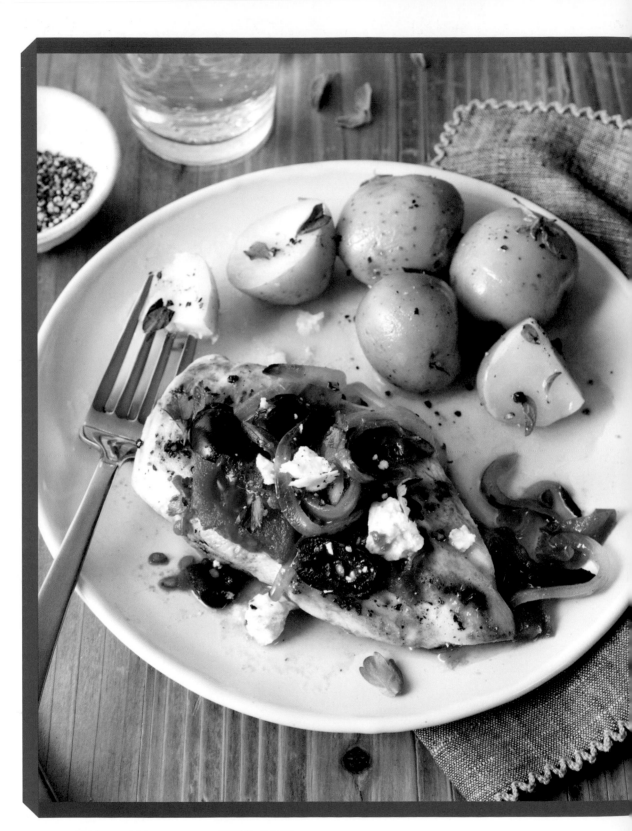

Greek-Style Chicken Breasts

Cooking spray

4   (6-ounce) skinless, boneless chicken breast halves
¼   teaspoon kosher salt
¼   teaspoon freshly ground black pepper
1½ tablespoons olive oil
1¾ cups vertically sliced onion
1   tablespoon minced garlic
1   ounce chopped pitted kalamata olives (about 14)
1   medium tomato, halved and sliced
¼   cup chopped fresh flat-leaf parsley
2   teaspoons chopped fresh oregano
2   teaspoons fresh lemon juice
1   ounce feta cheese, crumbled (about ¼ cup)

1. Heat a grill pan over medium-high heat. Coat pan with cooking spray. Sprinkle chicken with salt and pepper. Add chicken to pan; cook 6 minutes on each side or until done.
2. Heat a large skillet over medium-high heat. Add oil to pan; swirl to coat. Add onion and garlic; sauté 4 minutes. Add olives and tomato; cook 3 minutes or until tomato begins to break down, stirring occasionally. Remove pan from heat; stir in parsley, oregano, and juice. Top chicken with tomato and olive mixture; sprinkle feta over chicken.

YIELD | SERVES 4 (SERVING SIZE: 1 CHICKEN BREAST HALF, ABOUT ⅓ CUP TOMATO MIXTURE, AND ABOUT 1 TABLESPOON FETA)

CALORIES 311; FAT 13.2g (sat 3g, mono 6.8g, poly 1.5g); PROTEIN 38g; CARB 8g; FIBER 2g; CHOL 115mg; IRON 1mg; SODIUM 518mg; CALC 74mg

Chicken Verde Enchiladas

How do you shred chicken superfast? Insert two forks into the meat while it's still warm. Then pull apart to shred.

- ¾ cup chopped onion
- ¾ cup gluten-free unsalted chicken stock
- ½ cup salsa verde
- ⅓ cup finely chopped cilantro stems
- 2 tablespoons sliced pickled jalapeño pepper
- 5 teaspoons gluten-free all-purpose flour
- ½ teaspoon ground cumin
- 2 garlic cloves, thinly sliced
- 8 ounces shredded skinless, boneless rotisserie chicken breast (about 2 cups)
- ¾ cup chopped tomato
- 3 tablespoons reduced-fat sour cream
- 1 ripe peeled avocado, coarsely mashed
- 8 (6-inch) corn tortillas
- 4 ounces reduced-fat sharp cheddar cheese, shaved (about 1 cup)
- 2 tablespoons cilantro leaves

1. Position oven rack in lower third of oven, and preheat broiler.
2. Combine first 8 ingredients in a medium saucepan, stirring with a whisk. Bring to a boil; reduce heat, and simmer 4 minutes. Stir in chicken; cook 1 minute or until heated. Remove from heat. Stir in tomato, sour cream, and avocado.
3. Stack tortillas; wrap stack in damp paper towels, and microwave at HIGH 45 seconds. Spoon 1 cup chicken mixture into an 11 x 7–inch glass or ceramic baking dish. Spoon ⅓ cup chicken mixture in center of each tortilla; roll up. Arrange tortillas, seam sides down, in baking dish. Top with cheese. Broil 3 minutes or until cheese melts. Sprinkle with cilantro leaves.

YIELD | SERVES 4 (SERVING SIZE: 2 ENCHILADAS)

CALORIES 400; FAT 18g (sat 6.5g, mono 7.9g, poly 2g); PROTEIN 29g; CARB 33g; FIBER 7g; CHOL 75mg; IRON 1mg; SODIUM 620mg; CALC 267mg

Braised Chicken with Honey-Lemon Leeks

Lemon is a bright partner for the caramelized leeks, which cook twice: They are sautéed, then roasted to meld with the honey and lemon.

4	teaspoons olive oil, divided
8	bone-in, skinless chicken thighs (about 2 pounds)
¾	teaspoon kosher salt, divided
½	teaspoon freshly ground black pepper
1	tablespoon grated lemon rind
4	cups thinly sliced leek (about 3 large)
3	tablespoons fresh lemon juice
2	teaspoons honey
2	tablespoons chopped fresh parsley or chives (optional)

1. Preheat oven to 400°.

2. Heat a large ovenproof skillet over medium heat. Add 2 teaspoons oil to pan; swirl to coat. Sprinkle chicken with ½ teaspoon salt and pepper. Massage lemon rind into chicken. Place chicken in pan; cook 4 minutes on each side or until browned. Remove chicken from pan; keep warm.

3. Add 2 teaspoons oil to pan; swirl to coat. Add leek and ¼ teaspoon salt; cook 15 minutes or until leek begins to brown, scraping pan to loosen browned bits. Remove pan from heat; stir in juice and honey. Return chicken to pan. Mound leeks on top of chicken thighs. Bake chicken at 400° for 15 minutes or until a thermometer registers 165°. Top with fresh parsley or chives, if desired.

YIELD | SERVES 4 (SERVING SIZE: 2 THIGHS AND ABOUT ¼ CUP LEEK MIXTURE)

CALORIES 339; FAT 15.6g (sat 3.6g, mono 7.7g, poly 2.8g); PROTEIN 33g; CARB 17g; FIBER 2g; CHOL 175mg; IRON 4mg; SODIUM 492mg; CALC 72mg

Grilled Chicken Thighs with Cilantro-Mint Chutney

3   tablespoons grated fresh onion
½   teaspoon ground red pepper
10   garlic cloves, minced
2½   tablespoons canola oil, divided
2   teaspoons ground cumin, divided
4   (6-ounce) bone-in chicken thighs
½   teaspoon kosher salt, divided
Cooking spray
1   cup cilantro leaves
½   cup mint leaves
⅓   cup chopped green onions
2   teaspoons chopped seeded jalapeño pepper

1. Combine first 3 ingredients in a large zip-top plastic bag; stir in 2 tablespoons oil and 1¾ teaspoons cumin. Add chicken to bag, seal, and massage marinade into chicken. Marinate in refrigerator 2 hours.
2. Preheat grill to medium-high heat.
3. Remove chicken from bag. Sprinkle chicken with ¼ teaspoon salt. Place on grill rack coated with cooking spray; grill 8 minutes on each side.
4. Place cilantro, mint, green onions, and jalapeño in a food processor; process until combined. Add 1½ teaspoons oil, ¼ teaspoon cumin, and ¼ teaspoon salt; process until smooth. Serve chicken topped with chutney.

YIELD | SERVES 4 (SERVING SIZE: 1 THIGH AND ABOUT 1½ TABLESPOONS CHUTNEY)

CALORIES 331; **FAT** 24g (sat 4.8g, mono 11.8g, poly 5.5g); **PROTEIN** 24g; **CARB** 5g; **FIBER** 1g; **CHOL** 135mg; **IRON** 2mg; **SODIUM** 332mg; **CALC** 46mg

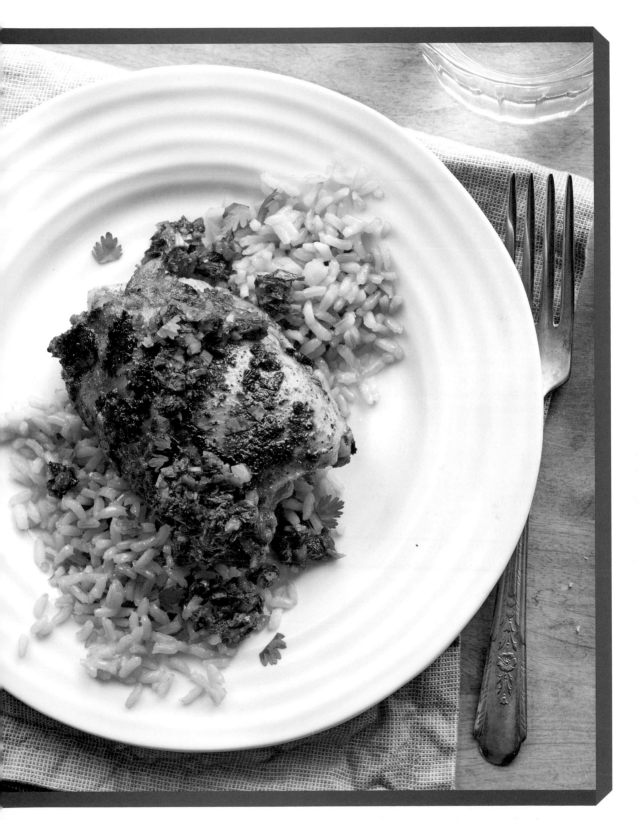

Dijon-Herb Chicken Thighs

2   tablespoons chopped fresh flat-leaf parsley
2   tablespoons chopped fresh chives
2   tablespoons olive oil
2   teaspoons Dijon mustard
2   garlic cloves, minced
4   (6-ounce) bone-in chicken thighs (about 1½ pounds), skinned
½   teaspoon kosher salt
½   teaspoon freshly ground black pepper
Cooking spray

1. Preheat oven to 450°.
2. Combine parsley, chives, olive oil, Dijon mustard, and garlic in a small bowl, stirring well with a whisk. Rub herb mixture over meaty side of chicken thighs; sprinkle with salt and pepper.
3. Arrange chicken on a baking sheet or jelly-roll pan coated with cooking spray. Bake at 450° for 25 minutes or until done.
4. Preheat broiler (do not remove pan from oven). Broil chicken 3 minutes or until browned.

YIELD | SERVES 4 (SERVING SIZE: 1 THIGH)

CALORIES 270; FAT 13.9g (sat 2.7g, mono 7.4g, poly 2.3g); PROTEIN 33g; CARB 1g; FIBER 0g; CHOL 162mg; IRON 2mg; SODIUM 453mg; CALC 23mg

Five-Bean Chili

Serving this chili the next day lets flavors meld—if the beans soak up a lot of liquid overnight, you can add more vegetable broth or even water to thin it out.

1	tablespoon canola oil
2	cups chopped onion
1	cup chopped carrot
2	tablespoons unsalted tomato paste
2	tablespoons minced fresh garlic
1½	teaspoons dried oregano
1½	teaspoons chili powder
1	teaspoon kosher salt
½	teaspoon Spanish smoked paprika
4	cups stemmed and torn kale
3	cups gluten-free organic vegetable broth
2	red bell peppers, chopped
1	jalapeño pepper, seeded and chopped
1	(16-ounce) can unsalted pinto beans, rinsed and drained
1	(15.8-ounce) can unsalted Great Northern beans, rinsed and drained
1	(15.5-ounce) can unsalted chickpeas (garbanzo beans), rinsed and drained
1	(15-ounce) can unsalted black beans, rinsed and drained
1	(15-ounce) can unsalted kidney beans, rinsed and drained
1	(14.5-ounce) can unsalted diced tomatoes, undrained

1. Heat a large Dutch oven over medium heat. Add oil; swirl to coat. Add onion and carrot; sauté 10 minutes or until tender. Stir in tomato paste and next 5 ingredients (through paprika); cook 2 minutes, stirring constantly. Add kale and remaining ingredients. Cover and simmer 45 minutes.

YIELD | SERVES 8 (SERVING SIZE: ABOUT 1½ CUPS)

CALORIES 221; FAT 2.8g (sat 0.2g, mono 1.2g, poly 0.7g); PROTEIN 11g; CARB 39g; FIBER 12g; CHOL 0mg; IRON 3mg; SODIUM 520mg; CALC 153mg

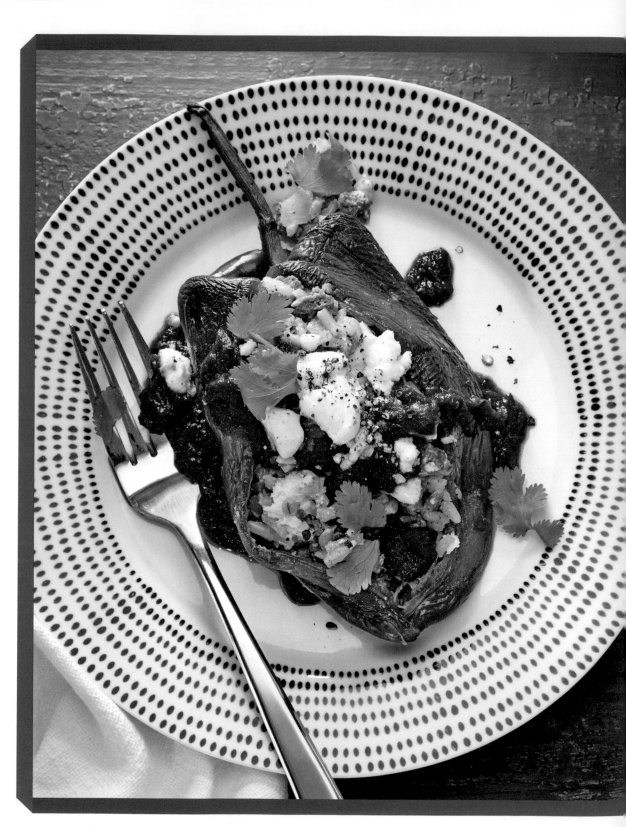

Stuffed Poblanos

 8 large poblano peppers
 4 dried ancho chiles
 2 tablespoons canola oil
 3 cups chopped onion
10 garlic cloves, minced
12 ounces ground sirloin
 1 teaspoon kosher salt, divided
 1 teaspoon black pepper
 4 ounces ⅓-less-fat cream cheese, softened (about ½ cup)
1½ cups precooked brown rice (such as Uncle Ben's Ready Rice)
 6 ounces queso fresco, crumbled and divided (about 1½ cups)
 ¼ cup fresh lime juice
 1 tablespoon ground cumin
 2 teaspoons sugar
 2 (14.5-ounce) cans unsalted diced tomatoes, undrained
    Cooking spray
 ¼ cup cilantro leaves

1. Preheat broiler.

2. Place poblanos on a foil-lined baking sheet; broil 3 inches from heat 12 minutes or until black-ened, turning after 6 minutes. Place in a paper bag; fold to close tightly. Let stand 15 minutes. Peel and discard skins. Cut a lengthwise slit in each pepper; discard seeds and membranes. Set aside.

3. Place ancho chiles in a bowl. Cover with boiling water; let stand 10 minutes. Drain.

4. Reduce oven temperature to 400°.

5. Heat a large skillet over medium heat. Add oil to pan; swirl. Add onion and garlic; cook 4 minutes or until crisp-tender. Reserve half of onion mixture. Add beef, ½ teaspoon salt, and black pepper; cook 8 minutes or until beef is done. Remove from heat. Add cream cheese, stirring until well combined. Stir in rice and half of queso fresco.

6. Place ancho chiles, reserved onion mixture, juice, cumin, sugar, tomatoes, and ½ teaspoon salt in a blender; process until smooth. Pour 1 cup sauce into each of 2 (8-inch) square glass or ceramic baking dishes coated with cooking spray. Open each poblano chile; flatten slightly. Divide beef mixture among chiles (they will be full). Arrange 4 chiles in each dish; top with remaining sauce and queso. Bake at 400° for 20 minutes or until bubbly. Sprinkle with cilantro.

YIELD | SERVES 8 (SERVING SIZE: 1 STUFFED CHILE AND ABOUT ⅔ CUP SAUCE)

CALORIES 334; FAT 14.8g (sat 5.2g, mono 5.5g, poly 1.8g); PROTEIN 18g; CARB 35g; FIBER 7g; CHOL 45mg; IRON 4mg; SODIUM 369mg; CALC 148mg

INGREDIENT TIP

Too hot? Poblano peppers range in heat level from quite spicy to rather mild, and there's no way to know what you're getting until you take a bite. If your peppers are too hot, cool off with a dollop of sour cream.

Sausage Pizza

2	teaspoons granulated sugar
1	package dry yeast (about 2¼ teaspoons)
½	cup warm water (100° to 110°)
3.65	ounces white rice flour (about ¾ cup)
1.4	ounces sweet white sorghum flour (about ⅓ cup)
1.4	ounces tapioca flour (about ⅓ cup)
1.7	ounces potato starch (about ⅓ cup)
0.9	ounce flaxseed meal (about ¼ cup)
1	teaspoon xanthan gum
¼	teaspoon salt
1	tablespoon olive oil
2	large egg whites
1	large egg
	Cooking spray
4	ounces turkey Italian sausage (1 link)
½	cup gluten-free, lower-sodium marinara sauce
4	ounces part-skim mozzarella cheese, shredded (about 1 cup)
2	tablespoons chopped ripe olives

1. Dissolve sugar and yeast in ½ cup warm water in a bowl; let stand 5 minutes.

2. Weigh or lightly spoon flours, potato starch, and flaxseed meal into dry measuring cups; level with a knife. Combine flours, potato starch, flaxseed meal, xanthan gum, and salt in a bowl; beat with a mixer at medium speed until blended. Add yeast mixture, oil, egg whites, and egg; beat at low speed until combined. Increase speed to medium; beat 2 minutes.

3. Spoon dough onto an 11 x 17–inch baking sheet coated with cooking spray and lined with parchment paper. Lightly coat hands with cooking spray; press dough into an 11 x 12–inch rectangle. Cover with plastic wrap coated with cooking spray, and let rise in a warm place (85°), free from drafts, 30 minutes.

4. Preheat oven to 400°.

5. Remove plastic wrap. Bake at 400° for 14 minutes or until bottom is crisp. Cool completely. Increase oven temperature to 425°.

6. Remove casing from sausage. Heat a large skillet over medium-high heat. Add sausage; cook 3 minutes. Spread marinara over crust, leaving a ½-inch border; top with sausage, cheese, and olives. Bake at 425° for 12 minutes or until golden.

YIELD | SERVES 6 (SERVING SIZE: 1 RECTANGLE)

CALORIES 309; FAT 11.8g (sat 3.6g, mono 4.7g, poly 2.2g); PROTEIN 15g; CARB 37g; FIBER 3.5g; CHOL 63mg; IRON 1.3mg; SODIUM 564mg; CALC 19mg

Vegetarian Lasagna

9   uncooked gluten-free lasagna noodles
1   teaspoon olive oil
7   cups sliced mushrooms
3   cups sliced shiitake mushroom caps
½   teaspoon ground nutmeg
3   garlic cloves, minced
6   tablespoons grated fresh Parmesan cheese, divided
1   teaspoon dried Italian seasoning
1   teaspoon freshly ground black pepper
3   large egg whites
2   (15-ounce) cartons part-skim ricotta cheese
2   (10-ounce) packages frozen chopped spinach, thawed, drained, and squeezed dry
1   (25.5-ounce) jar gluten-free marinara sauce
    Cooking spray
12 ounces shredded part-skim mozzarella cheese, divided (about 3 cups)

1. Cook lasagna noodles according to package directions, omitting salt and fat. Drain; set aside.

2. Heat oil in a nonstick skillet over medium heat. Add mushrooms; sauté 3 minutes. Add nutmeg and garlic; sauté 5 minutes. Set aside.

3. Combine ¼ cup Parmesan cheese, Italian seasoning, pepper, egg whites, ricotta, and spinach; set aside.

4. Preheat oven to 375°.

5. Spread ½ cup marinara sauce in bottom of a 13 x 9–inch glass or ceramic baking dish coated with cooking spray. Arrange 3 lasagna noodles over sauce; top with half of ricotta cheese mixture, half of mushroom mixture, 1½ cups sauce, and 1 cup mozzarella cheese. Repeat layers, ending with noodles. Spread ½ cup sauce over noodles.

6. Cover and bake at 375° for 40 minutes. Uncover; sprinkle with 1 cup mozzarella cheese and 2 tablespoons Parmesan cheese; bake 10 minutes. Let stand 10 minutes before serving.

YIELD | SERVES 9

CALORIES 430; FAT 17g (sat 10.1g, mono 2.8g, poly 0.5g); PROTEIN 30g; CARB 39g; FIBER 4g; CHOL 52mg; IRON 3mg; SODIUM 741mg; CALC 661mg

Three-Cheese Baked Penne

Since gluten-free pasta can clump and stick together if it stands for a while, be sure to cook it al dente (since it'll cook a bit more while it bakes), and have it ready just in time to toss with the sauce.

- 2 teaspoons olive oil
- 1½ cups finely chopped onion (about 1 medium)
- 1 (12-ounce) package gluten-free brown rice penne
- 4 cups 1% low-fat milk or dairy-free alternative, divided
- ¼ cup cornstarch
- ¾ teaspoon salt
- ½ teaspoon freshly ground black pepper
- ½ teaspoon grated whole nutmeg
- 4 ounces reduced-fat sharp cheddar cheese, shredded (about 1 cup)
- 4 ounces shredded part-skim mozzarella cheese (about 1 cup)
- Cooking spray
- 2 ounces grated fresh Parmesan cheese (about ½ cup)
- ¼ cup gluten-free panko (Japanese breadcrumbs)

1. Preheat oven to 375°.

2. Heat oil in a medium Dutch oven over medium heat. Add onion; cook 5 minutes or until tender, stirring often.

3. While onion cooks, cook pasta according to package directions, omitting salt and fat. Drain.

4. Combine ½ cup milk and cornstarch in a small bowl. Add 3½ cups milk to onion; bring to a boil. Gradually stir in cornstarch mixture. Cook 2 minutes or until sauce thickens, stirring constantly. Remove from heat, and stir in salt, pepper, and nutmeg. Add cheddar and mozzarella cheeses, stirring with a whisk until cheeses melt. Stir in pasta. Pour pasta mixture into 6 (2-cup) gratin dishes or ramekins coated with cooking spray. Combine Parmesan cheese and panko; sprinkle over pasta mixture. Bake at 375° for 30 minutes or until sauce is bubbly and top is brown.

YIELD | SERVES 6 (SERVING SIZE: ABOUT 1¼ CUPS)

CALORIES 493; FAT 14.5g (sat 7.7g, mono 3.4g, poly 0.5g); PROTEIN 23g; CARB 67g; FIBER 2g; CHOL 40mg; IRON 4mg; SODIUM 308mg; CALC 767mg

Tomato-Basil Pasta with Asiago

2	cups (6 ounces) uncooked gluten-free rice penne
¾	cup canned unsalted navy beans, rinsed and drained
2	tablespoons extra-virgin olive oil
1	cup grape tomatoes, halved
¼	cup finely chopped green onions
½	teaspoon minced fresh rosemary
12	pitted kalamata olives, coarsely chopped
2	garlic cloves, minced
2	cups fresh baby spinach, coarsely chopped
3	ounces grated Asiago cheese (about ¾ cup)
¼	cup chopped fresh basil
½	teaspoon salt
½	teaspoon freshly ground black pepper

1. Cook pasta according to package directions, omitting salt and fat; add beans during last 1 minute of cooking. Drain pasta and beans, reserving ¼ cup pasta water. Place pasta, beans, and reserved pasta water in a large shallow pasta bowl.

2. While pasta cooks, heat oil in a medium nonstick skillet over medium heat. Add tomatoes; cook 2 minutes, stirring often. Stir in green onions and next 3 ingredients (through garlic); cook 2 minutes or just until tomatoes are thoroughly heated. Remove from heat.

3. Add spinach and next 4 ingredients (through pepper) to pasta mixture. Toss well. Top with tomato mixture.

YIELD | SERVES 4 (SERVING SIZE: 1⅓ CUPS)

CALORIES 394; FAT 17.4g (sat 5.2g, mono 7.7g, poly 1g); PROTEIN 11g; CARB 48g; FIBER 5g; CHOL 19mg; IRON 4mg; SODIUM 718mg; CALC 243mg

INGREDIENT TIP
Fresh rosemary

You can easily strip rosemary leaves from their tough, inedible stems by holding the top of a stem in one hand, and then pulling in the opposite direction of the way the leaves grow. You can substitute ½ teaspoon crushed dried rosemary for the fresh, if you'd like.

Pasta with Roasted Red Pepper and Cream Sauce

1	pound uncooked gluten-free seashell pasta
2	teaspoons extra-virgin olive oil
½	cup finely chopped onion
1	(12-ounce) bottle roasted red bell peppers, drained and coarsely chopped
2	teaspoons balsamic vinegar
1	cup half-and-half
1	tablespoon tomato paste
⅛	teaspoon ground red pepper
4	ounces grated fresh Parmigiano-Reggiano cheese, divided (about 1 cup)

Thinly sliced fresh basil (optional)

1. Cook pasta according to package directions, omitting salt and fat. Drain and keep warm.

2. Heat oil in a large skillet over medium heat. Add onion, and cook 8 minutes or until tender, stirring frequently. Add bell peppers; cook 2 minutes or until thoroughly heated. Increase heat to medium-high. Stir in vinegar; cook 1 minute or until liquid evaporates. Remove from heat; cool 5 minutes.

3. Place bell pepper mixture in a blender; process until smooth. Return bell pepper mixture to pan; cook over low heat until warm. Combine half-and-half and tomato paste in a small bowl, stirring with a whisk. Stir tomato mixture into bell pepper mixture, stirring with a whisk until well combined. Stir in ground red pepper.

4. Combine pasta and bell pepper mixture in a large bowl. Add ½ cup cheese, tossing to coat. Spoon 1⅓ cups pasta into each of 6 bowls; top each serving with about 1½ tablespoons cheese. Garnish with basil, if desired.

YIELD | SERVES 6

CALORIES 442; FAT 12.3g (sat 6.4g, mono 2.8g, poly 0.4g); PROTEIN 14g; CARB 67g; FIBER 0g; CHOL 32mg; IRON 5mg; SODIUM 422mg; CALC 305mg

Pasta Carbonara Florentine

6   center-cut bacon slices, chopped
1   cup finely chopped onion
2   tablespoons dry white wine
1   (6-ounce) package bagged prewashed baby spinach
8   ounces uncooked gluten-free spaghetti
2   ounces grated fresh Parmesan cheese (about ½ cup)
½   teaspoon salt
½   teaspoon freshly ground black pepper
1   large egg
1   large egg white
3   tablespoons chopped fresh parsley

1. Heat a large nonstick skillet over medium heat. Add bacon to pan; cook 5 minutes or until crisp, stirring frequently. Remove bacon from pan, reserving 2 teaspoons drippings in pan; set bacon aside.
2. Add onion to drippings in pan; cook 3 minutes or until tender, stirring frequently. Add wine; cook 1 minute or until liquid is reduced by half. Add spinach; cook 1 minute or until spinach wilts, stirring constantly. Remove from heat; keep warm.
3. Cook pasta according to package directions, omitting salt and fat. Drain well, reserving 1 tablespoon pasta water. Immediately add pasta and reserved pasta water to spinach mixture in pan. Add reserved bacon; stir well to combine. Place pan over low heat.
4. Combine cheese and next 4 ingredients (through egg white), stirring with a whisk. Add to pasta mixture, tossing well to coat. Cook 1 minute. Remove from heat. Sprinkle with parsley. Serve immediately.

YIELD | SERVES 4 (SERVING SIZE: 1 CUP)

CALORIES 373; FAT 9.8g (sat 4.3g, mono 2.5g, poly 0.5g); PROTEIN 16g; CARB 55g; FIBER 3g; CHOL 72mg; IRON 6mg; SODIUM 773mg; CALC 257mg

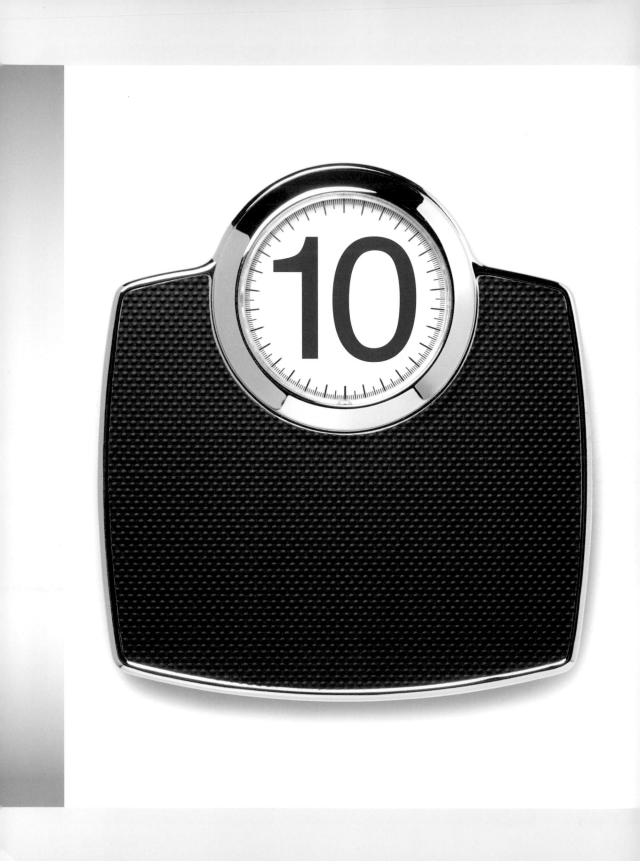

SNACKS ARE A CRUCIAL COMPONENT OF ANY DIET. Keeping healthy snacks on hand that work with your meal plan is key to keeping hunger at bay. Use these snacks and sides to hold you over between meals and round out your plate.

Roasted Garlic and Chive Dip

Serve with sweet mini bell peppers or sliced summer squash. If you can find roasted garlic cloves at the salad bar in your grocery store, sub for raw garlic and skip the 8 minutes of cooking in the skillet.

- ½ cup unpeeled garlic cloves
- ½ cup plain fat-free Greek yogurt
- ½ cup light sour cream
- 2 tablespoons minced fresh chives
- ⅜ teaspoon salt
- Dash of freshly ground black pepper

1. Heat a large nonstick skillet over medium heat. Add garlic cloves to pan; cover and cook 8 minutes or until lightly browned and tender when pierced with a fork, stirring occasionally. Cool slightly. Squeeze garlic from skins into the bowl of a mini food processor. Discard skins. Puree garlic until smooth.

2. Combine yogurt, sour cream, chives, salt, and pepper in a medium bowl, stirring well with a whisk. Add garlic to yogurt mixture, stirring with a whisk to combine.

YIELD | SERVES 8 (SERVING SIZE: ABOUT 2 TABLESPOONS)

CALORIES 42; FAT 1.7g (sat 1g, mono 0.5g, poly 0.1g); PROTEIN 2g; CARB 5g; FIBER 0g; CHOL 5mg; IRON 0mg; SODIUM 128mg; CALC 47mg

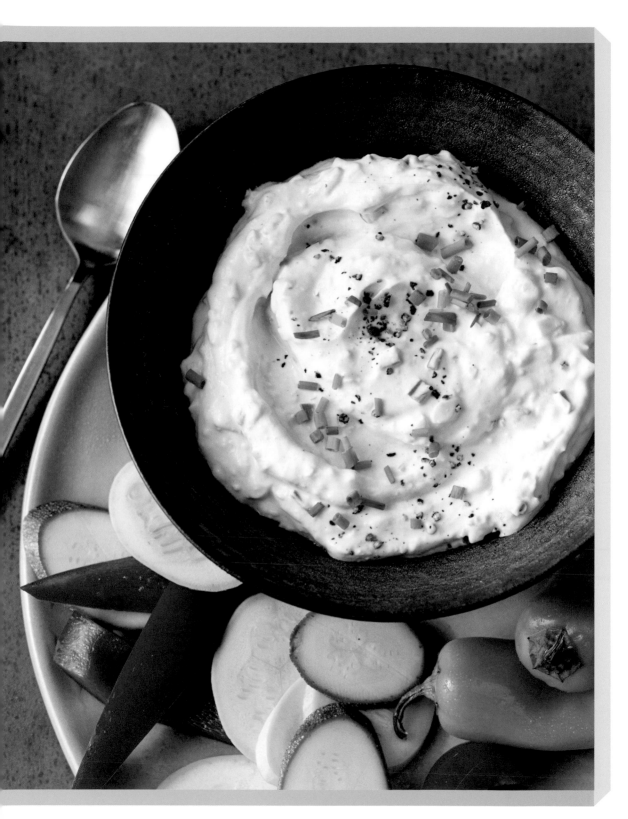

Cheddar-Bacon-Chive Dip

5   **tablespoons fat-free sour cream**
1   **tablespoon canola mayonnaise**
3   **tablespoons finely shredded cheddar cheese**
2   **tablespoons finely chopped chives**
2   **slices cooked and crumbled center-cut bacon**
Dash of freshly ground black pepper
2   **ounces reduced-fat kettle-cooked potato chips**

1. Combine sour cream, mayonnaise, cheese, chives, bacon, and black pepper. Serve with potato chips.

YIELD | SERVES 4 (SERVING SIZE: ½ OUNCE POTATO CHIPS [ABOUT 10 CHIPS] AND ABOUT 2 TABLESPOONS DIP)

CALORIES 128; FAT 7g (sat 2g, mono 3.4g, poly 0.9g); PROTEIN 4g; CARB 13g; FIBER 1g; CHOL 11mg; IRON 0mg; SODIUM 223mg; CALC 68mg

Green Goodness Dip

This dip is a riff on the classic green goddess dressing. It's made thicker with a base of pureed peas enriched with Greek yogurt and creamy avocado. Serve it with assorted fresh vegetables.

1	cup fresh or frozen green peas, thawed
1	cup plain fat-free Greek yogurt
½	cup flat-leaf parsley leaves
3	tablespoons chopped fresh chives
2	tablespoons fresh lemon juice
1	tablespoon chopped fresh tarragon
½	teaspoon kosher salt
¼	teaspoon freshly ground black pepper
3	canned anchovy fillets, drained
½	ripe peeled avocado

1. Combine all ingredients in a food processor; process until smooth.

YIELD | SERVES 8 (SERVING SIZE: ¼ CUP)

CALORIES 54; FAT 2.1g (sat 0.3g, mono 1.3g, poly 0.3g); PROTEIN 4g; CARB 5g; FIBER 2g; CHOL 1mg; IRON 1mg; SODIUM 207mg; CALC 35mg

Mozza Fruit Skewers

1	part-skim mozzarella cheese stick	8	grapes
4	pineapple chunks	2	skewers
4	strawberry halves		

1. Cut cheese stick into 4 pieces. Thread cheese, pineapple chunks, strawberry halves, and grapes onto skewers.

YIELD | SERVES 1

CALORIES 97; FAT 1.7g (sat 1g, mono 0.2g, poly 0.1g); PROTEIN 9g; CARB 13g; FIBER 1g; CHOL 5mg; IRON 0mg; SODIUM 221mg; CALC 211mg

Edamame Crunch

For the late-night munchies, try this snack. It packs in 11 grams of protein in a half-cup serving. Try it sautéed or roasted, too.

| ½ | cup shelled edamame | Dash of kosher salt |
| 1 | teaspoon toasted sesame seeds | |

1. Boil shelled edamame in water to cover until crisp-tender. Sprinkle with toasted sesame seeds and a dash of kosher salt.

YIELD | SERVES 1

CALORIES 117; FAT 4g (sat 0.2g, mono 0.6g, poly 0.7g); PROTEIN 11g; CARB 10g; FIBER 1g; CHOL 0mg; IRON 2mg; SODIUM 190mg; CALC 109mg

Lemon-Parmesan Popcorn

To make sure the oil is ready for the popcorn, add a couple of kernels and wait for them to pop. Once they pop, add the remaining kernels.

- 2 teaspoons grated lemon rind
- 1 teaspoon freshly ground black pepper
- ¼ teaspoon kosher salt
- 1.5 ounces Parmigiano-Reggiano cheese, finely grated (about ⅓ cup)
- 2 tablespoons olive oil
- ½ cup unpopped popcorn kernels

1. Combine lemon rind, pepper, salt, and cheese in a small bowl.

2. Heat oil in a medium, heavy saucepan over medium-high heat. Add popcorn to oil in pan; cover and cook 2 minutes or until kernels begin to pop, shaking pan frequently. Continue cooking 1 minute, shaking pan constantly. When popping slows to a couple seconds between pops, remove pan from heat. Let stand 1 minute or until all popping stops. Pour 6 cups popcorn into a large bowl; stir in half of cheese mixture. Stir in remaining 6 cups popcorn and remaining half of cheese mixture; toss to coat. Let stand 1 minute before serving.

YIELD | SERVES 6 (SERVING SIZE: 2 CUPS)

CALORIES 128; FAT 7.2g (sat 1.9g, mono 3.9g, poly 0.6g); PROTEIN 4g; CARB 12g; FIBER 3g; CHOL 6mg; IRON 1mg; SODIUM 189mg; CALC 81mg

Pan-Charred Asparagus

Toasted walnuts lend a delightful nutty crunch to this asparagus. It's a quick and easy side and a nice change from roasted asparagus.

Cooking spray

8 ounces (2½-inch) pieces trimmed asparagus

1½ teaspoons toasted walnut oil

2 teaspoons lemon juice

2 teaspoons chopped fresh tarragon

¼ teaspoon kosher salt

2 tablespoons shaved Parmigiano-Reggiano cheese

1 tablespoon chopped toasted walnuts

1. Heat a medium, heavy skillet (not nonstick) over high heat 2 minutes.

2. Coat pan with cooking spray. Immediately add asparagus pieces to pan, shaking them into a single layer; cook, without stirring, 2 minutes or until asparagus is very lightly charred. Cook asparagus 5 minutes or until crisp-tender and evenly charred, tossing occasionally.

3. Remove pan from heat. Let asparagus rest 1 minute. Add walnut oil; toss to coat asparagus pieces. Add lemon juice; toss. Turn on heat if necessary to evaporate most of liquid. Sprinkle asparagus with tarragon and salt; toss. Sprinkle with cheese and walnuts. Serve immediately.

YIELD | SERVES 4 (SERVING SIZE: ABOUT ⅔ CUP)

CALORIES 52; FAT 4g (sat 0.7g, mono 0.8g, poly 2.2g); PROTEIN 3g; CARB 3g; FIBER 1g; CHOL 2mg; IRON 1mg; SODIUM 160mg; CALC 45mg

Browned Butter and Lemon Brussels Sprouts

1½	pounds Brussels sprouts, trimmed and halved	¼	teaspoon kosher salt
¼	cup water	¼	teaspoon freshly ground black pepper
2	tablespoons unsalted butter	1	teaspoon grated lemon rind
		1	tablespoon fresh lemon juice

1½ pounds Brussels sprouts, trimmed and halved
¼ cup water
2 tablespoons unsalted butter
¼ teaspoon kosher salt
¼ teaspoon freshly ground black pepper
1 teaspoon grated lemon rind
1 tablespoon fresh lemon juice

1. Heat a large skillet over medium-high heat. Add Brussels sprouts and ¼ cup water to pan; cover and cook 5 minutes. Add butter, salt, and pepper to pan; cook, uncovered, 2 minutes. Increase heat to high; cook 1 minute, stirring frequently. Stir in lemon rind and lemon juice.

YIELD | SERVES 6 (SERVING SIZE: ABOUT ⅔ CUP)

CALORIES 84; FAT 4.2g (sat 2.5g, mono 1g, poly 0.3g); PROTEIN 4g; CARB 10g; FIBER 4g; CHOL 10mg; IRON 2mg; SODIUM 109mg; CALC 50mg

Cabbage Slaw with Mango Vinaigrette

½ cup chopped mango
1 tablespoon canola oil
1 tablespoon fresh lime juice
¼ teaspoon salt
5 cups thinly sliced green cabbage
½ cup diced mango
¼ cup thinly sliced green onions
3 tablespoons chopped toasted cashews

1. Combine chopped mango, canola oil, lime juice, and salt in a mini food processor; process until smooth. Place cabbage, diced mango, and green onions in a large bowl, tossing to combine. Drizzle cabbage mixture with pureed mango mixture; toss to coat. Sprinkle with cashews.

YIELD | SERVES 6 (SERVING SIZE: ABOUT ¾ CUP)

CALORIES 79; FAT 4.5g (sat 0.6g, mono 2.7g, poly 1g); PROTEIN 2g; CARB 9g; FIBER 2g; CHOL 0mg; IRON 1mg; SODIUM 110mg; CALC 32mg

Sautéed Green Beans with Spice-Glazed Pecans

The glazed pecans can be made up to three days in advance and stored in an airtight container at room temperature. Double the recipe to have some on hand for easy snacks.

2	tablespoons sugar
1	tablespoon water
¼	teaspoon ground cumin
¼	teaspoon ground red pepper
¾	cup coarsely chopped pecans
1	teaspoon minced fresh rosemary
½	teaspoon kosher salt, divided
2	pounds green beans, trimmed
2	tablespoons unsalted butter
¼	teaspoon freshly ground black pepper

1. Preheat oven to 350°. Line a jelly-roll pan with parchment paper.

2. Bring sugar, 1 tablespoon water, cumin, and red pepper to a boil in a small saucepan over medium heat, stirring constantly until sugar dissolves. Remove pan from heat; stir in pecans, rosemary, and ¼ teaspoon salt. Spread pecan mixture in an even layer on prepared pan. Bake at 350° for 12 minutes or until fragrant and browned. Cool in pan, stirring occasionally.

3. Place green beans in a large saucepan of boiling water; cook 4 minutes. Drain and plunge green beans into ice water; drain.

4. Melt butter in a nonstick skillet over medium-high heat. Add beans; sauté 5 minutes or until heated. Sprinkle ¼ teaspoon salt and black pepper over beans; toss. Place beans on a serving platter; sprinkle with pecan mixture. Serve immediately.

YIELD | SERVES 12 (SERVING SIZE: ¾ CUP)

CALORIES 96; FAT 7g (sat 1.7g, mono 3.3g, poly 1.6g); PROTEIN 2g; CARB 8g; FIBER 3g; CHOL 5mg; IRON 1mg; SODIUM 85mg; CALC 34mg

Caprese Zucchini

Cooking spray
2 medium zucchini, sliced
½ cup diced seeded tomato
2 tablespoons chopped fresh basil
2 teaspoons olive oil

1 teaspoon red wine vinegar
¼ teaspoon kosher salt
¼ teaspoon freshly ground black pepper
1 ounce shredded part-skim
   mozzarella cheese (about ¼ cup)

1. Heat a grill pan over medium-high heat. Coat pan with cooking spray. Grill zucchini slices 2 minutes on each side.

2. Preheat broiler.

3. Combine tomato, basil, olive oil, vinegar, salt, and pepper. Arrange grilled zucchini on a foil-lined baking sheet; top with tomato mixture and mozzarella. Broil 2 minutes or until cheese melts.

YIELD | SERVES 4 (SERVING SIZE: 4 ZUCCHINI SLICES, 2 TABLESPOONS TOMATO MIXTURE, AND 1 TABLESPOON CHEESE)

CALORIES 64; FAT 4.2g (sat 1.2g, mono 2g, poly 0.4g); PROTEIN 3g; CARB 4g; FIBER 1g; CHOL 4mg; IRON 1mg; SODIUM 175mg; CALC 72mg

Beet–Blood Orange Salad

1½ pounds halved peeled beets
1   blood orange
2   tablespoons toasted walnut oil
2   tablespoons minced shallots
½   teaspoon Dijon mustard
¼   teaspoon freshly ground black pepper

⅛   teaspoon salt
2   cups mixed greens
⅓   cup chopped unsalted,
    dry-roasted pistachios
2   tablespoons goat cheese

1. Wrap beets in parchment paper. Microwave at HIGH until tender (about 7 minutes). Let stand 5 minutes. Cut into 1-inch pieces.

2. Section orange over a bowl; squeeze to juice. Place sections in a bowl. Add oil, shallots, mustard, pepper, and salt to juice; stir. Add beets, greens, and orange sections; toss. Top with pistachios and cheese.

YIELD | SERVES 4 (SERVING SIZE: ABOUT ¾ CUP)

CALORIES 229; FAT 12.3g (sat 1.7g, mono 4g, poly 5.8g); PROTEIN 6g; CARB 26g; FIBER 7g; CHOL 3mg; IRON 2mg; SODIUM 247mg; CALC 58mg

Bourbon Baked Beans

Check your beans 10 to 15 minutes ahead of time to make sure they're not drying out.

1	pound dried navy beans (about 2½ cups)
3	applewood-smoked bacon slices
1	cup finely chopped onion
5	cups water, divided
½	cup maple syrup, divided
¼	cup plus 2 tablespoons bourbon, divided
¼	cup Dijon mustard
1½	teaspoons gluten-free Worcestershire sauce
¼	teaspoon freshly ground black pepper
1	tablespoon cider vinegar
1	teaspoon salt

1. Sort and wash beans; place in a large Dutch oven. Cover with water to 2 inches above beans; cover and let stand 8 hours or overnight. Drain beans. Wipe pan dry with a paper towel.
2. Preheat oven to 350°.
3. Heat pan over medium-high heat. Add bacon to pan, and cook 4 minutes or until crisp. Remove bacon from pan, reserving 1½ tablespoons drippings in pan; crumble bacon. Add onion to drippings in pan; cook 5 minutes or until onion begins to brown, stirring frequently. Add beans, bacon, 4 cups water, ¼ cup maple syrup, ¼ cup bourbon, and next 3 ingredients (through pepper) to pan. Bring to a boil; cover and bake at 350° for 2 hours.
4. Stir in 1 cup water, ¼ cup maple syrup, and 2 tablespoons bourbon. Cover and bake 1 hour or until beans are tender and liquid is almost absorbed. Stir in vinegar and salt.

YIELD | SERVES 13 (SERVING SIZE: ½ CUP)

CALORIES 199; FAT 3.1g (sat 1.1g, mono 0.7g, poly 0.5g); PROTEIN 8g; CARB 32g; FIBER 6g; CHOL 4mg; IRON 2mg; SODIUM 307mg; CALC 66mg

Simmered Pinto Beans with Chipotle Sour Cream

Refried beans can be high in fat; instead, serve these pinto beans simmered with earthy cumin.

2   teaspoons olive oil
½   cup chopped onion
½   cup chopped red bell pepper
½   teaspoon ground cumin
2   garlic cloves, minced
½   cup gluten-free unsalted chicken stock
⅛   teaspoon kosher salt
⅛   teaspoon freshly ground black pepper
1   (15-ounce) can unsalted pinto beans, rinsed and drained
1   tablespoon lemon juice
2   tablespoons chopped fresh flat-leaf parsley
¾   cup reduced-fat sour cream
3   tablespoons low-fat buttermilk
1½   teaspoons minced chipotle chiles, canned in adobo sauce

1. Heat a saucepan over medium-high heat. Add oil; swirl to coat. Add onion, bell pepper, cumin, and garlic; sauté 2 minutes. Add stock, salt, black pepper, and beans; simmer 7 minutes. Stir in juice and parsley.
2. Combine sour cream, buttermilk, and chiles; serve with beans.

YIELD | SERVES 6 (SERVING SIZE: ABOUT ¼ CUP BEANS AND 2 TABLESPOONS CREAM)

CALORIES 128; FAT 5.4g (sat 2.6g, mono 1.1g, poly 0.2g); PROTEIN 5g; CARB 14g; FIBER 4g; CHOL 16mg; IRON 1mg; SODIUM 100mg; CALC 99mg

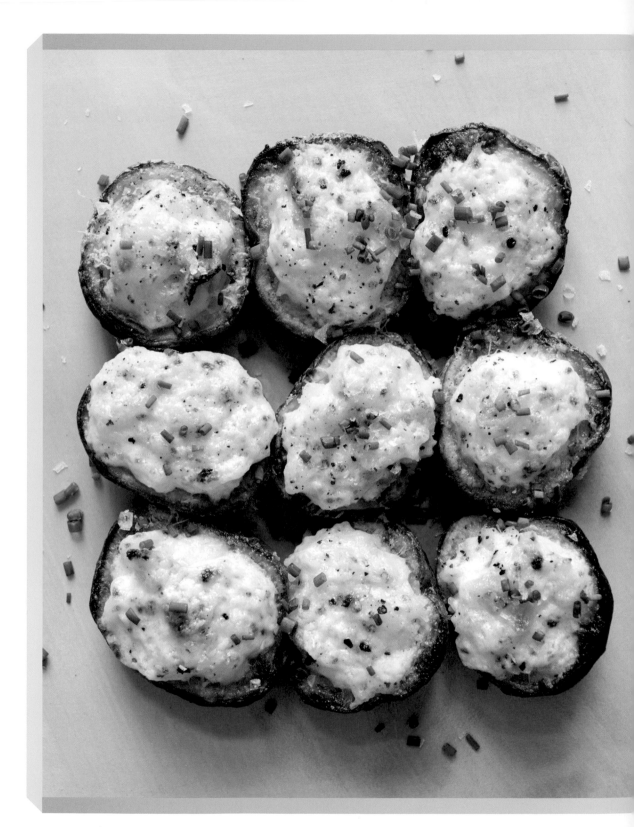

Lemon-Caper Parmesan Potato Salad Bites

Turn "jacket potatoes" into irresistible potato salad bites.
Capers offer a twist on traditional relish; they're actually pickled
flower buds and add bright, briny flavor to this appetizer.

12	small red potatoes, halved (about 1¼ pounds)
2	teaspoons olive oil
½	cup light sour cream
2	tablespoons minced fresh chives, divided
2	tablespoons butter, melted
2	tablespoons finely chopped drained capers
1½	teaspoons lemon juice
½	teaspoon kosher salt
½	teaspoon freshly ground black pepper
2	tablespoons grated Parmesan cheese

1. Preheat oven to 450°.

2. Combine potatoes and oil; toss to coat. Arrange potatoes, cut sides down, in a single layer on a parchment paper–lined baking sheet. Bake at 450° for 20 minutes. Turn potatoes; bake 10 minutes. Remove and cool 20 minutes.

3. Preheat broiler.

4. Using a paring knife, carefully cut a circle in cut side of potatoes. Using a melon baller or small spoon, remove pulp from potato, leaving a thin shell. Combine pulp, sour cream, 1 tablespoon chives, and next 5 ingredients (through pepper). Fill potato shells with filling; sprinkle with cheese and 1 tablespoon chives.

5. Broil potatoes 2 minutes or until cheese is lightly browned.

YIELD | SERVES 12 (SERVING SIZE: 2 POTATO HALVES)

CALORIES 85; FAT 3.9g (sat 2.2g, mono 1.2g, poly 0.2g); PROTEIN 2g; CARB 10g; FIBER 1g; CHOL 6mg; IRON 0mg; SODIUM 182mg; CALC 20mg

Pan-Seared Mojo Potatoes

4   teaspoons olive oil, divided
1   pound fingerling potatoes, halved lengthwise
⅜   teaspoon salt
⅔   cup tightly packed cilantro
2   teaspoons lime juice
1   teaspoon white wine vinegar
¼   teaspoon black pepper
1   large garlic clove, chopped
¼   cup reduced-fat sour cream

1. Heat a skillet over medium-high heat. Add 1 tablespoon oil and potatoes; cook 6 minutes. Cover, reduce heat to medium, and cook 6 minutes.
2. Sprinkle potatoes with salt. Combine 1 teaspoon oil, cilantro, and next 4 ingredients (through garlic) in a blender. Blend until smooth. Stir into potatoes. Top with sour cream.

YIELD | SERVES 4

CALORIES 151; FAT 6.5g (sat 1.8g, mono 3.3g, poly 0.5g); PROTEIN 4g; CARB 20g; FIBER 2g; CHOL 8mg; IRON 1mg; SODIUM 280mg; CALC 44mg

Goat Cheese and Basil Polenta

3	cups water	1	tablespoon chopped fresh basil
1	cup dry polenta	¼	teaspoon freshly ground black pepper
3	ounces goat cheese (about ⅓ cup)	¼	teaspoon kosher salt

1. Bring 3 cups water to a boil in a medium saucepan. Gradually add polenta, stirring constantly with a whisk. Reduce heat to low; cook 7 minutes, stirring occasionally. Remove from heat; stir in goat cheese, basil, pepper, and salt.

YIELD | SERVES 4 (SERVING SIZE: ¾ CUP)

CALORIES 204; FAT 4.5g (sat 3.1g, mono 1g, poly 0.1g); PROTEIN 7g; CARB 32g; FIBER 1g; CHOL 10mg; IRON 2mg; SODIUM 198mg; CALC 32mg

Rustic Garlic Mashed Potatoes

2	pounds unpeeled baking potatoes, quartered lengthwise	1½	tablespoons butter, melted
1	garlic head, peeled	½	teaspoon salt
¾	cup hot 1% low-fat milk or dairy-free alternative	¼	teaspoon freshly ground black pepper

1. Place potatoes and garlic head in a saucepan filled with water to cover; bring to a boil. Reduce heat, and simmer 15 minutes or until potatoes are tender. Drain and transfer to a bowl; mash with hot milk, butter, salt, and pepper.

YIELD | SERVES 4 (SERVING SIZE: ABOUT 1 CUP)

CALORIES 259; FAT 5g (sat 3.1g, mono 1.3g, poly 0.3g); PROTEIN 7g; CARB 48g; FIBER 3g; CHOL 14mg; IRON 2mg; SODIUM 363mg; CALC 116mg

Garlic-Parmesan Rice

1	tablespoon olive oil	¼	teaspoon kosher salt
1	garlic clove, minced	⅛	teaspoon black pepper
1	cup uncooked basmati rice	1	ounce grated fresh Parmesan cheese (about ¼ cup)
2	cups water		
1	tablespoon chopped fresh flat-leaf parsley		

1. Heat a saucepan over medium heat. Add oil to pan. Add garlic; sauté 30 seconds. Add rice; cook 1 minute, stirring constantly. Add 2 cups water; bring to a boil. Cover, reduce heat, and simmer 12 minutes or until liquid is absorbed. Remove from heat. Let stand 5 minutes. Stir in parsley, salt, pepper, and cheese.

YIELD | SERVES 4 (SERVING SIZE: ABOUT ¾ CUP)

CALORIES 242; FAT 5.4g (sat 1.7g, mono 3.1g, poly 0.4g); PROTEIN 5g; CARB 46g; FIBER 1g; CHOL 6mg; IRON 2mg; SODIUM 229mg; CALC 82mg

Wild Rice with Squash

5	cups water	1	teaspoon chopped fresh rosemary
⅔	cup uncooked wild rice	⅜	teaspoon salt, divided
1½	tablespoons olive oil	1	shallot, chopped
1½	cups (½-inch) cubed peeled butternut squash	⅛	teaspoon freshly ground black pepper

1. Place 5 cups water and rice in a saucepan; bring to a boil. Cover, reduce heat, and simmer 30 minutes. Turn off heat; let stand, covered, 25 minutes. Drain. Heat a skillet over medium heat; add oil. Add squash, rosemary, ⅛ teaspoon salt, and shallot; cook 10 minutes. Add rice, pepper, and ¼ teaspoon salt to squash mixture, stirring to combine.

YIELD | SERVES 4 (SERVING SIZE: ABOUT 1 CUP)

CALORIES 169; FAT 5.4g (sat 0.8g, mono 3.7g, poly 0.7g); PROTEIN 5g; CARB 27g; FIBER 3g; CHOL 0mg; IRON 1mg; SODIUM 185mg; CALC 34mg

Yogurt Rice with Cumin and Chile

Using whole packages of rice and yogurt saves the time of measuring. Be sure to use standard yogurt here; Greek is a bit too thick. Serve with grilled lamb chops, roasted chicken, or grilled salmon.

2 (8.5-ounce) pouches precooked white basmati rice (such as Uncle Ben's)
1 tablespoon canola oil
1 tablespoon bottled minced fresh ginger
1 teaspoon cumin seeds
1 serrano chile, thinly sliced
2 tablespoons chopped fresh cilantro
¾ teaspoon kosher salt
1 (6-ounce) carton plain low-fat yogurt

1. Heat rice according to package directions.
2. Heat a large skillet over medium-high heat. Add oil; swirl to coat. Add ginger, cumin, and chile; sauté 30 seconds. Stir in rice, cilantro, salt, and yogurt; cook 1 minute.

YIELD | SERVES 6 (SERVING SIZE: ½ CUP)

CALORIES 173; FAT 4.6g (sat 0.8g, mono 2.1g, poly 1.4g); PROTEIN 5g; CARB 29g; FIBER 1g; CHOL 2mg; IRON 1mg; SODIUM 265mg; CALC 56mg

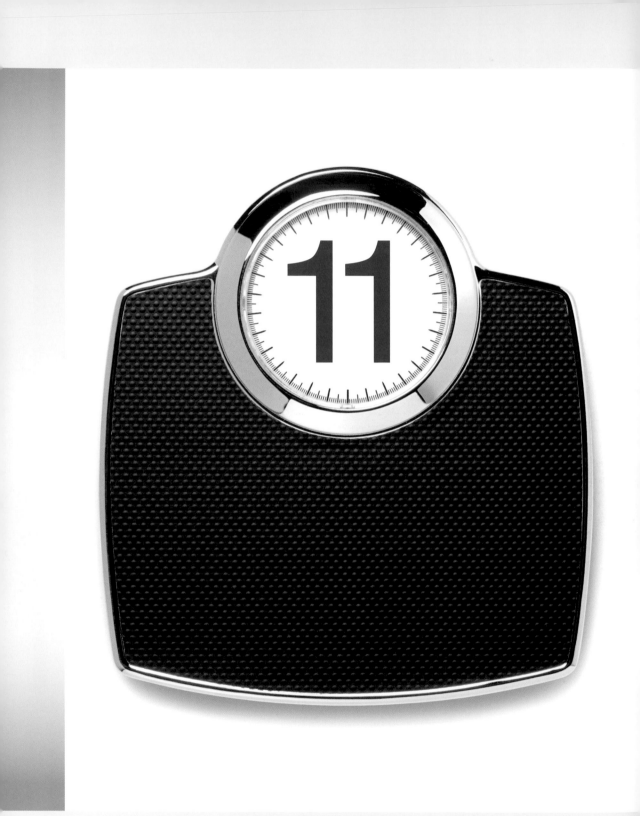

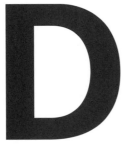

D

ESSERT IS AN IMPORTANT PART OF ANY DIET, INCLUDING THIS ONE. While something sweet doesn't need to be part of every meal, satisfying your cravings will actually help keep you on track with your weight loss. These recipes offer healthier options that don't have the excess calories and saturated fat that many ready-made gluten-free desserts do. Just remember that moderation is key.

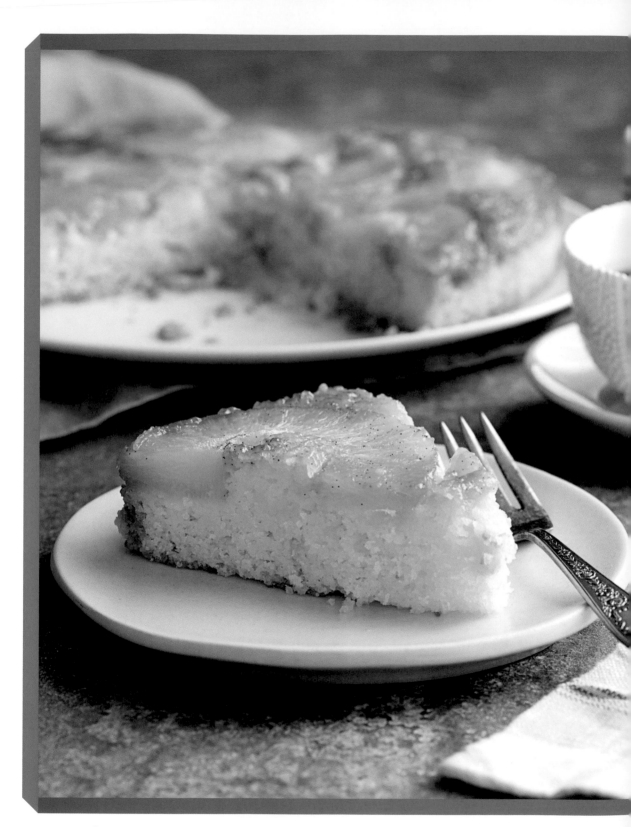

Pineapple Upside-Down Cake

½   cup packed brown sugar

¼   cup unsalted butter, divided

1   vanilla bean, split lengthwise

6   (½-inch-thick) slices fresh pineapple

¼   cup dark rum

Cooking spray

5   ounces gluten-free all-purpose flour (about 1 cup)

0.9 ounces almond meal flour (about ¼ cup)

½   teaspoon baking powder

½   teaspoon kosher salt

¼   teaspoon baking soda

½   cup light sour cream

2   tablespoons canola oil

⅔   cup granulated sugar

2   large eggs

1. Preheat oven to 350°.

2. Combine brown sugar, 2 tablespoons butter, and vanilla bean in a skillet over medium heat; cook 6 minutes or until butter melts and sugar dissolves, stirring frequently. Add pineapple in a single layer. Carefully pour rum over pineapple; tilt pan to ignite. Simmer 5 minutes on each side or until slightly tender and caramelized. Remove vanilla bean.

3. Coat a 9-inch round cake pan with cooking spray. Arrange pineapple in a single layer in bottom of pan; pour sugar mixture over pineapple, tilting pan to coat bottom.

4. Weigh or lightly spoon flours into dry measuring cups; level with a knife. Combine flours, baking powder, salt, and baking soda. Melt 2 tablespoons butter in a microwave-safe dish at HIGH 35 seconds. Combine melted butter, sour cream, and oil in a bowl.

5. Beat granulated sugar and eggs with a mixer at high speed 5 minutes or until fluffy. Reduce speed to medium. Add flour mixture and sour cream mixture alternately to egg mixture, beginning and ending with flour mixture. Spread batter over pineapple. Bake at 350° for 38 minutes or until a wooden pick inserted in center comes out clean. Cool in pan 15 minutes on a wire rack.

YIELD | SERVES 10 (SERVING SIZE: 1 WEDGE)

CALORIES 292; **FAT** 11.2g (sat 4.4g, mono 3.7g, poly 1.2g); **PROTEIN** 4g; **CARB** 44g; **FIBER** 1g; **CHOL** 54mg; **IRON** 1mg; **SODIUM** 177mg; **CALC** 87mg

INGREDIENT TIP

Cooking with alcohol

The rum will ignite when you tilt the pan; this burns off most of the alcohol but leaves a delicious flavor behind.

Cocoa Cupcakes

2.1 ounces sweet white sorghum flour (about ½ cup)

1.15 ounces brown rice flour (about ¼ cup)

1.05 ounces tapioca flour (about ¼ cup)

½ cup unsweetened cocoa

1 teaspoon xanthan gum

½ teaspoon baking soda

½ teaspoon baking powder

½ teaspoon salt

¾ cup granulated sugar

¼ cup unsalted butter, softened

2 large eggs

1 cup fat-free sour cream

½ teaspoon vanilla extract

Cooking spray

1 cup powdered sugar

2 tablespoons unsalted butter, softened

1 tablespoon 1% low-fat milk

½ teaspoon vanilla extract

1. Preheat oven to 375°.

2. Weigh or lightly spoon flours into dry measuring cups; level with a knife. Combine flours, cocoa, and next 4 ingredients (through salt) in a medium bowl; stir with a whisk.

3. Place granulated sugar and ¼ cup butter in a large bowl; beat with a mixer at medium speed until blended. Add eggs, 1 at a time, beating well after each addition. Beat in sour cream and ½ teaspoon vanilla. Gradually add flour mixture, beating at low speed until smooth (batter will be very thick).

4. Place 12 paper muffin cup liners in muffin cups; coat liners with cooking spray. Spoon batter into prepared cups (cups will be almost full). Bake at 375° for 20 minutes or until a wooden pick inserted in center comes out clean. Cool in pan 10 minutes on a wire rack; remove from pan. Cool completely on wire rack.

5. Combine powdered sugar, 2 tablespoons butter, milk, and ½ teaspoon vanilla in a medium bowl; beat with a mixer at low speed until blended. Increase speed to medium; beat until smooth. Spread frosting over cupcakes.

YIELD | SERVES 12 (SERVING SIZE: 1 CUPCAKE)

CALORIES 218; FAT 7.7g (sat 4.4g, mono 2.1g, poly 0.4g); PROTEIN 4g; CARB 36g; FIBER 2g; CHOL 48mg; IRON 1mg; SODIUM 199mg; CALC 57mg

Blackberry-Almond Cobbler

4   cups fresh blackberries
3   tablespoons sugar
1   tablespoon cornstarch
1   tablespoon fresh lemon juice
Cooking spray
2.3 ounces brown rice flour (about ½ cup)
1.8 ounces almond meal flour (about ½ cup)
¼   cup sugar
1   teaspoon baking powder
⅛   teaspoon salt
1   large egg, beaten
4   tablespoons butter, melted and cooled
2   cups vanilla light ice cream

1. Preheat oven to 375°.
2. Place blackberries in a large bowl; add 3 tablespoons sugar, cornstarch, and juice, stirring to coat berries. Pour mixture into an 8-inch square glass or ceramic baking dish coated with cooking spray.
3. Weigh or lightly spoon flours into dry measuring cups; level with a knife. Combine flours, ¼ cup sugar, baking powder, and salt in a large bowl, stirring with a whisk. Add egg, stirring to combine. Add butter, stirring just until moist.
4. Drop batter by teaspoonfuls onto blackberry mixture. Bake at 375° for 30 minutes or until topping is lightly browned. Cool 10 minutes. Serve with ice cream.

YIELD | SERVES 8 (SERVING SIZE: ⅛ OF COBBLER AND ¼ CUP ICE CREAM)

CALORIES 276; FAT 12.2g (sat 5.3g, mono 2.5g, poly 0.7g); PROTEIN 6g; CARB 38g; FIBER 5g; CHOL 49mg; IRON 1mg; SODIUM 183mg; CALC 143mg

Grilled Peaches with Honey Cream

You can use apricots or nectarines instead of peaches.

2   tablespoons unsalted butter, melted
2   tablespoons honey, divided
¼   teaspoon ground cardamom
Dash of kosher salt
4   medium peaches, pitted and halved
Cooking spray
⅓   cup plain fat-free Greek yogurt
2½   tablespoons half-and-half
¼   teaspoon vanilla extract
1   cup raspberries
Mint leaves (optional)

1. Combine butter, 1 tablespoon honey, cardamom, and salt in a medium bowl. Add peaches, and toss to coat. Let stand 5 minutes.

2. Heat a grill pan over medium heat. Coat pan with cooking spray. Arrange peaches on grill pan; grill 2 minutes on each side or until grill marks appear.

3. Combine yogurt, half-and-half, 1 tablespoon honey, and vanilla in a small bowl; stir with a whisk. Serve with peaches and raspberries. Garnish with mint leaves, if desired.

YIELD | SERVES 4 (SERVING SIZE: 2 PEACH HALVES, ¼ CUP RASPBERRIES, AND 2 TABLESPOONS YOGURT MIXTURE)

CALORIES 182; FAT 7.6g (sat 4.4g, mono 1.6g, poly 0.5g); PROTEIN 4g; CARB 28g; FIBER 4g; CHOL 19mg; IRON 1mg; SODIUM 43mg; CALC 42mg

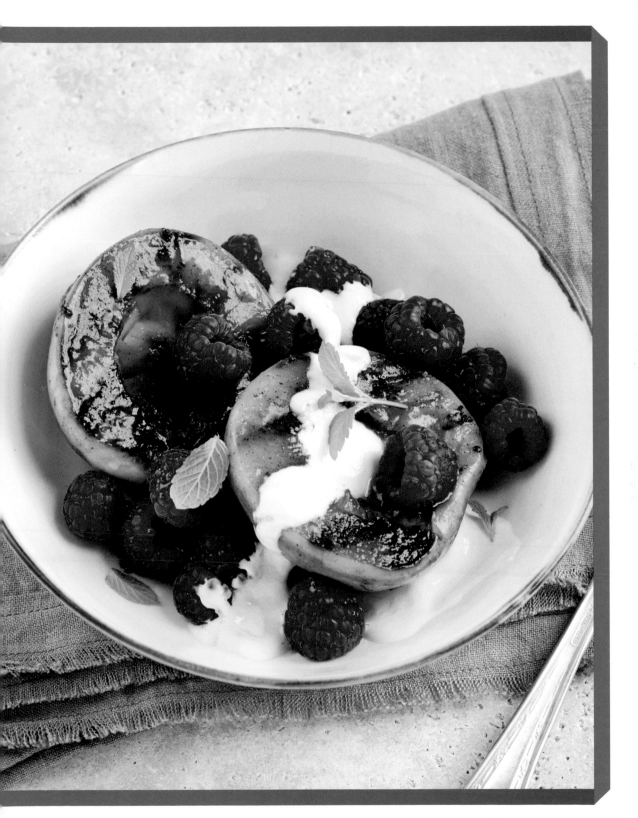

Meyer Lemon Panna Cotta

Meyer lemon—a lemon/orange hybrid—is sweeter than conventional lemon. If you don't have access to Meyer lemons, you can use a regular lemon and enjoy a dessert that's a bit more tart.

1	**Meyer or regular lemon**
½	**cup plus 3 tablespoons 2% reduced-fat milk, divided**
½	**cup half-and-half**
⅓	**cup sugar**
¼	**teaspoon salt**
1¾	**teaspoons unflavored gelatin**
1½	**cups low-fat buttermilk**
	Cooking spray
	Mint leaves and lemon rind strips (optional)

1. Remove rind from lemon using a vegetable peeler, avoiding white pith. Squeeze 3 tablespoons juice from lemon. Combine rind, ½ cup reduced-fat milk, half-and-half, sugar, and salt in a small saucepan; bring to a simmer over medium heat (do not boil). Remove pan from heat; cover and let stand 20 minutes. Discard rind. Sprinkle gelatin over 3 tablespoons reduced-fat milk in a small bowl, and let stand at least 10 minutes.

2. Return half-and-half mixture to medium heat; cook 1 minute or until very hot. Add gelatin mixture, stirring with a whisk until dissolved (about 1 minute). Stir in buttermilk and 3 tablespoons juice. Divide mixture among 4 (6-ounce) ramekins or custard cups coated with cooking spray. Cover and refrigerate 4 hours.

3. Run a knife around outside edges of each panna cotta. Place a plate upside down on top of each cup; invert panna cotta onto plate. Garnish with mint and lemon rind strips, if desired.

YIELD | SERVES 4

CALORIES 185; FAT 6.3g (sat 3.8g, mono 0.8g, poly 0.1g); PROTEIN 7g; CARB 26g; FIBER 0g; CHOL 22mg; IRON 0mg; SODIUM 258mg; CALC 214mg

Chocolate–Peanut Butter Pudding

⅓ cup sugar

2 tablespoons cornstarch

2 tablespoons Dutch process cocoa

1½ cups 1% low-fat milk

½ cup light cream

2 ounces milk chocolate, finely chopped

¼ cup creamy peanut butter

1 tablespoon chopped unsalted, dry-roasted peanuts

1. Combine sugar, cornstarch, and cocoa in a medium saucepan; stir with a whisk. Whisk in milk and cream. Bring to a boil over medium-high heat. Cook 1 minute or until thick and bubbly. Remove from heat. Add chocolate and peanut butter, stirring until smooth. Spoon about ⅓ cup pudding into each of 6 bowls. Top each serving with ½ teaspoon peanuts.

YIELD | SERVES 6

CALORIES 245; FAT 13.7g (sat 5.4g, mono 3.8g, poly 1.9g); PROTEIN 6g; CARB 27g; FIBER 1g; CHOL 12mg; IRON 1mg; SODIUM 104mg; CALC 123mg

Butterscotch Pudding

½ cup packed dark brown sugar

3½ tablespoons cornstarch

⅛ teaspoon salt

2 cups 1% low-fat milk

2 large egg yolks, lightly beaten

1 tablespoon butter

2 teaspoons vanilla extract

Cooking spray

5 teaspoons almond brickle chips (such as Heath)

1. Combine brown sugar, cornstarch, and salt in a medium saucepan over medium heat. Add milk and egg yolks, stirring with a whisk until smooth.
2. Bring mixture to a boil, and cook 2 to 3 minutes or until mixture thickens, stirring constantly.
3. Remove pan from heat; stir in butter and vanilla. Pour mixture into 5 (6-ounce) ramekins or small bowls. Cover surface of pudding with plastic wrap coated with cooking spray; cool 15 minutes. Chill at least 4 hours. Top each serving with 1 teaspoon brickle chips.

YIELD | SERVES 5

CALORIES 220; FAT 6.6g (sat 3.4g, mono 1.7g, poly 0.4g); PROTEIN 5g; CARB 35g; FIBER 0g; CHOL 86mg; IRON 0mg; SODIUM 152mg; CALC 150mg

Jasmine Chai Rice Pudding

Although it keeps several days in the fridge, this pudding is at its best warm. Add a touch of extra milk to reheat, and top with whipped topping, nuts, and rind just before serving.

2	cups 1% low-fat milk, divided
1½	cups water
2	teaspoons loose chai tea (about 4 tea bags)
⅛	teaspoon salt
1	cup uncooked jasmine rice
¾	cup sweetened condensed milk
¼	cup diced dried mixed fruit
2	large egg yolks
1	tablespoon butter
6	tablespoons frozen fat-free whipped topping, thawed
2	tablespoons chopped pistachios
½	teaspoon grated orange rind

1. Combine 1 cup low-fat milk, 1½ cups water, tea, and salt in a large saucepan; bring to a boil. Remove from heat; steep 1 minute. Strain milk mixture through a fine sieve into a bowl; discard solids. Return milk mixture to pan; place pan over medium heat. Stir in rice. Cover and simmer 10 minutes. Combine 1 cup low-fat milk, condensed milk, fruit, and egg yolks, stirring well with a whisk. Gradually add half of hot milk mixture to egg yolk mixture, stirring constantly with a whisk. Return milk mixture to pan; cook 10 minutes or until mixture is thick and rice is tender, stirring constantly. Remove from heat; stir in butter.

2. Place ⅔ cup rice pudding in each of 6 bowls. Top each serving with 1 tablespoon whipped topping. Combine nuts and rind. Sprinkle about 1 teaspoon nut mixture over each serving.

YIELD | SERVES 6

CALORIES 287; FAT 8.8g (sat 4.5g, mono 3g, poly 0.8g); PROTEIN 8g; CARB 44g; FIBER 1g; CHOL 90mg; IRON 1mg; SODIUM 169mg; CALC 223mg

Almond-Date Bars

Marcona almonds are blanched and roasted—you won't need to toast them. You can also substitute regular whole almonds. For the best texture, use whole pitted dates, not chopped; you need the sticky texture of the whole fruit.

1¼ cups pitted dates (about 15)
1   cup Marcona almonds
¾   cup dried apples (about 2 ounces)
¼   cup flaked sweetened coconut
1   tablespoon honey
⅛   teaspoon kosher salt
¾   cup crispy rice cereal
Cooking spray

1. Place first 6 ingredients in the bowl of a food processor; process until finely chopped. Add cereal; pulse to combine. Press date mixture into bottom of an 8-inch square glass or ceramic baking dish coated with cooking spray. Cut into 12 pieces.

YIELD | SERVES 12 (SERVING SIZE: 1 BAR)

CALORIES 142; FAT 6.3g (sat 1g, mono 3.7g, poly 1.5g); PROTEIN 3g; CARB 22g; FIBER 3g; CHOL 0mg; IRON 1mg; SODIUM 76mg; CALC 36mg

Maple-Pecan Bars

2.6 **ounces white rice flour (about ½ cup)**

2.3 **ounces cornstarch (about ½ cup)**

2.1 **ounces sweet sorghum flour (about ½ cup)**

½ **cup packed brown sugar**

6 **tablespoons butter**

1 **teaspoon xanthan gum**

2 **teaspoons vanilla extract**

¼ **teaspoon salt**

½ **cup maple syrup**

⅓ **cup packed brown sugar**

¼ **cup 1% low-fat milk**

1 **tablespoon butter**

½ **cup whole pecans**

½ **teaspoon vanilla extract**

1. Preheat oven to 375°. Line a 9-inch square metal baking pan with parchment paper.

2. Weigh or lightly spoon white rice flour, cornstarch, and sweet sorghum flour into dry measuring cups; level with a knife. Place white rice flour, cornstarch, sweet sorghum flour, ½ cup brown sugar, 6 tablespoons butter, xanthan gum, 2 teaspoons vanilla, and salt in a food processor; pulse until mixture resembles fine meal. Press flour mixture into bottom of prepared pan. Bake at 375° for 15 minutes or until edges of crust are lightly browned.

3. While crust bakes, combine syrup, ⅓ cup brown sugar, milk, and 1 tablespoon butter in a medium saucepan; bring to a boil over medium heat. Cook 2 minutes, stirring constantly with a whisk until sugar dissolves. Remove from heat; add pecans and ½ teaspoon vanilla, stirring with a whisk. Pour mixture into hot crust. Bake at 375° for 10 minutes or until filling is bubbly. Cool completely in pan. Cut into 20 bars.

YIELD | SERVES 20 (SERVING SIZE: 1 BAR)

CALORIES 149; FAT 6.2g (sat 2.8g, mono 2.2g, poly 0.8g); PROTEIN 1g; CARB 23g; FIBER 1g; CHOL 11mg; IRON 0mg; SODIUM 70mg; CALC 23mg

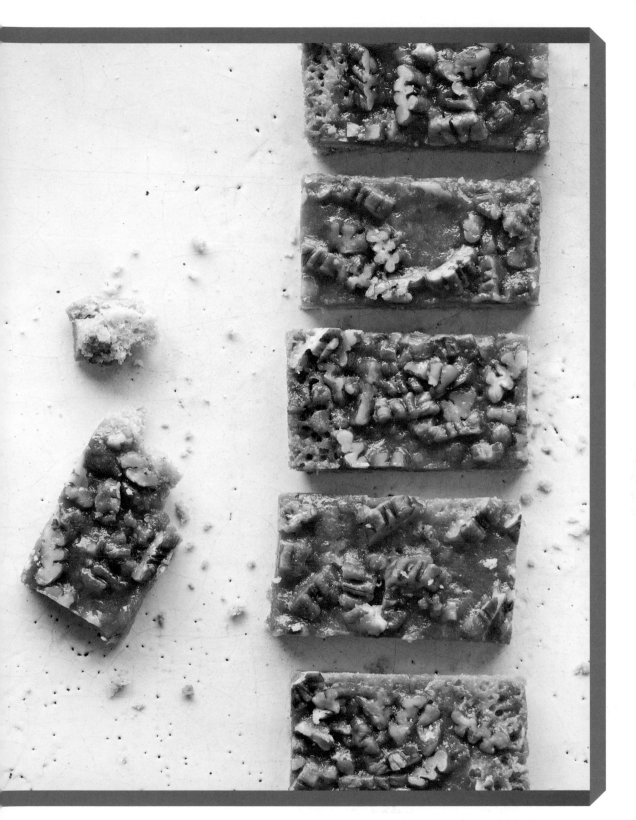

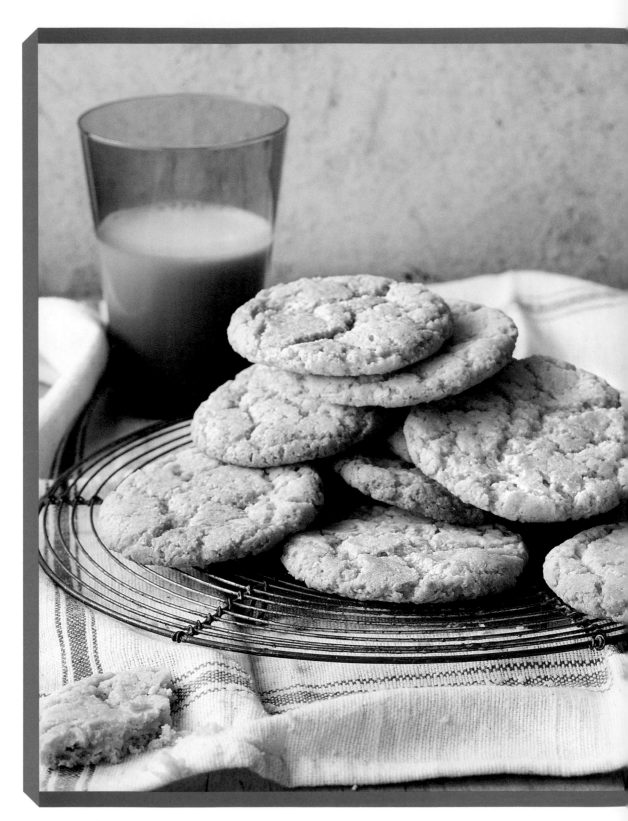

Lemon Sugar Cookies

The stark contrast between the sweet sugars and the tart lemon rind gives these cookies personality and bite. They're a great afternoon treat with coffee or tea.

2.3 ounces brown rice flour (about ½ cup)
1.8 ounces almond meal flour (about ½ cup)
1.05 ounces tapioca flour (about ¼ cup)
1.3 ounces potato starch (about ¼ cup)
1 teaspoon xanthan gum
1 teaspoon baking powder
¼ teaspoon salt
4 tablespoons butter, softened
½ cup granulated sugar
½ cup packed brown sugar
1 tablespoon fresh lemon juice
1 teaspoon vanilla extract
½ teaspoon grated lemon rind
2 large egg yolks

1. Preheat oven to 350°.
2. Weigh or lightly spoon flours and starch into dry measuring cups; level with a knife. Combine flours, potato starch, xanthan gum, baking powder, and salt in a medium bowl, stirring with a whisk.
3. Place butter and sugars in a bowl; beat with a mixer at medium speed until well blended. Add juice, vanilla, rind, and egg yolks; beat until blended. Add flour mixture, ¼ cup at a time, beating after each addition.
4. Cover a large baking sheet with parchment paper. Shape dough into 20 balls. Place 2 inches apart on baking sheet. Bake at 350° for 15 to 20 minutes or until lightly browned. Cool on pan 5 minutes. Remove cookies from pan; cool completely on wire racks.

YIELD | SERVES 20 (SERVING SIZE: 1 COOKIE)

CALORIES 105; FAT 4.1g (sat 1.7g, mono 0.8g, poly 0.2g); PROTEIN 1g; CARB 17g; FIBER 1g; CHOL 25mg; IRON 0mg; SODIUM 75mg; CALC 30mg

Peanut Butter–Chocolate Chip Cookies

You probably have everything on hand to make these chewy, chocolaty peanut butter cookies. To fit the cookies on a single sheet pan, divide cookies into five rows of four. Pressing the cookies flat helps them bake quickly and get lovely crisp edges; otherwise they'll be too round and undercooked.

- ¼ teaspoon salt
- 1 large egg white
- 1 cup reduced-fat chunky peanut butter
- ⅓ cup granulated sugar
- ¼ cup packed brown sugar
- ¼ cup semisweet chocolate minichips

1. Preheat oven to 375°.

2. Place salt and egg white in a medium bowl; stir with a whisk until white is frothy. Add peanut butter, granulated sugar, brown sugar, and chocolate chips, stirring to combine.

3. Divide dough into 20 equal portions (about 1 tablespoon each); arrange dough 2 inches apart on a baking sheet lined with parchment paper. Gently press the top of each cookie with a fork; press the top of each cookie again to form a crisscross pattern, and flatten to a 2-inch diameter. Bake at 375° for 10 minutes or until lightly browned.

YIELD | SERVES 20 (SERVING SIZE: 1 COOKIE)

CALORIES 111; FAT 5.6g (sat 1.4g, mono 2.6g, poly 1.4g); PROTEIN 3g; CARB 13g; FIBER 1g; CHOL 0mg; IRON 0mg; SODIUM 121mg; CALC 3mg

Amaretti

1	cup granulated sugar	2	large egg whites
1	(7-ounce) package almond paste	¼	cup turbinado sugar
1	teaspoon amaretto (almond-flavored liqueur)		

1. Preheat oven to 350°.

2. Place granulated sugar and almond paste in a large bowl; beat with a mixer at medium speed until almond paste is broken into small pieces. Add amaretto and egg whites; beat at high speed 4 minutes or until smooth. Chill batter 20 minutes.

3. Drop batter by teaspoonfuls 1 inch apart on parchment paper–lined baking sheets. Sprinkle with turbinado sugar. Bake at 350° for 10 minutes or until edges of cookies are golden brown. Cool completely on pans; carefully remove cookies from parchment. Cool on wire racks.

YIELD | SERVES 40 (SERVING SIZE: 1 COOKIE)

CALORIES 48; FAT 1.4g (sat 0.1g, mono 0.9g, poly 0.3g); PROTEIN 1g; CARB 9g; FIBER 0g; CHOL 0mg; IRON 0mg; SODIUM 3mg; CALC 9mg

Lemon Verbena–Buttermilk Sherbet

1	cup granulated sugar	2½	cups cold whole-milk buttermilk
¾	cup water	1	tablespoon grated lemon rind
3	tablespoons packed, coarsely chopped lemon verbena		Dash of salt
			Lemon rind strips (optional)

1. Combine first 3 ingredients in a saucepan, stirring until sugar dissolves. Bring to a boil; boil 2 minutes. Remove from heat; let stand 30 minutes. Pour syrup through a fine sieve into a bowl; discard solids. Stir in buttermilk, rind, and salt; chill 1 hour.

2. Pour mixture into the freezer can of an ice-cream freezer; freeze according to manufacturer's instructions. Spoon sherbet into a freezer-safe container; cover and freeze 1 hour or until firm. Garnish with lemon rind strips, if desired.

YIELD | SERVES 8 (SERVING SIZE: ABOUT ½ CUP)

CALORIES 145; FAT 2.5g (sat 1.5g, mono 0.6g, poly 0.2g); PROTEIN 2g; CARB 29g; FIBER 0g; CHOL 8mg; IRON 0mg; SODIUM 99mg; CALC 89mg

Cherry-Grapefruit-Basil Sorbet

1   cup water
½   cup sugar
Dash of kosher salt
½   cup basil leaves

3   cups pitted cherries
½   cup fresh ruby red grapefruit juice (about 1 grapefruit)
1½ teaspoons fresh lime juice

1. Combine first 3 ingredients in a small saucepan; bring to a boil, stirring until sugar dissolves. Stir in basil; remove from heat. Cover and let stand 30 minutes.

2. Place cherries in a food processor; process until smooth. Add syrup, grapefruit juice, and lime juice; process until well blended. Strain cherry mixture through a fine sieve over a bowl; discard solids. Pour cherry mixture into the freezer can of an ice-cream freezer; freeze according to manufacturer's instructions. Spoon sorbet into a freezer-safe container; cover and freeze 1 hour or until firm.

YIELD | SERVES 7 (SERVING SIZE: ½ CUP)

CALORIES 105; FAT 0.2g (sat 0g, mono 0g, poly 0.1g); PROTEIN 1g; CARB 27g; FIBER 1g; CHOL 0mg; IRON 0mg; SODIUM 18mg; CALC 16mg

Quick Berry Frozen Yogurt

2   cups frozen mixed berries, divided
1   cup vanilla low-fat frozen yogurt, divided

¼   cup fat-free milk
1   tablespoon chopped fresh mint
1   tablespoon honey

1. Combine 1 cup berries, ¾ cup yogurt, milk, mint, and honey in the bowl of a food processor; process until smooth. Spoon into a freezer-safe container. Add 1 cup berries and ¼ cup yogurt to processor; process until smooth. Swirl berry mixture into yogurt mixture. Serve immediately, or freeze until firm.

YIELD | SERVES 4 (SERVING SIZE: ABOUT ½ CUP)

CALORIES 150; FAT 2.5g (sat 1.3g, mono 0.4g, poly 0.2g); PROTEIN 6g; CARB 29g; FIBER 2g; CHOL 33mg; IRON 0mg; SODIUM 34mg; CALC 155mg

Blueberry Cheesecake Ice Cream

2	cups granulated sugar
6	ounces ⅓-less-fat cream cheese, softened (about ¾ cup)
4	large egg yolks
3	cups 2% reduced-fat milk
1	cup half-and-half
3	cups fresh blueberries, coarsely chopped
¼	cup powdered sugar
¼	cup water

1. Combine first 3 ingredients in a large bowl; beat with a mixer at high speed until smooth. Combine milk and half-and-half in a medium, heavy saucepan; bring to a boil. Remove from heat. Gradually add half of hot milk mixture to cheese mixture, stirring constantly with a whisk. Return milk mixture to pan. Cook over medium-low heat 5 minutes or until a thermometer registers 160°, stirring constantly. Place pan in an ice-filled bowl. Cool completely, stirring occasionally.

2. Combine blueberries, powdered sugar, and ¼ cup water in a small saucepan; bring to a boil. Reduce heat, and simmer 10 minutes or until mixture thickens slightly, stirring frequently. Remove from heat, and cool completely.

3. Stir blueberry mixture into milk mixture. Pour mixture into the freezer can of an ice-cream freezer; freeze according to manufacturer's instructions. Spoon ice cream into a freezer-safe container; cover and freeze 1 hour or until firm.

Note: This recipe yields 2 quarts of ice cream, so if you make the entire recipe, use a traditional bucket-style freezer. Halve the recipe if you use a countertop model; they typically have a smaller capacity.

YIELD | SERVES 12 (SERVING SIZE: ABOUT ⅔ CUP)

CALORIES 268; FAT 7.8g (sat 4.4g, mono 2.3g, poly 0.5g); PROTEIN 5g; CARB 46g; FIBER 1g; CHOL 90mg; IRON 0mg; SODIUM 100mg; CALC 49mg

Raspberries with Peach-Basil Sorbet

Here's a twist on peach Melba, the classic dessert of poached peaches with raspberry sauce. We turn juicy summer peaches instead into a velvety sorbet spiked with basil and serve it with fresh raspberries for the perfect ending to a summer meal.

1   cup granulated sugar
¾   cup water
¼   cup packed, coarsely chopped fresh basil leaves
1½   pounds ripe peaches
1   tablespoon fresh lemon juice
Dash of salt
12   ounces fresh raspberries
Basil sprigs (optional)

1. Combine first 3 ingredients in a saucepan. Bring to a boil; stir until sugar dissolves. Let stand 15 minutes. Pour through a fine sieve into a bowl; discard solids.
2. Cook peaches in a large pot of boiling water 1 minute. Place peaches in a bowl of ice water until cool. Peel peaches; remove pits and chop flesh. Place chopped peaches and juice in a blender; process until smooth. Stir peach mixture and salt into basil mixture. Chill 1 hour.
3. Pour peach mixture into the freezer can of an ice-cream freezer; freeze according to manufacturer's instructions. Spoon sorbet into a freezer-safe container; cover and freeze until firm. Serve with raspberries. Garnish with basil sprigs, if desired.

YIELD | SERVES 6 (SERVING SIZE: ½ CUP SORBET AND ABOUT ⅓ CUP RASPBERRIES)

CALORIES 199; FAT 0.6g (sat 0g, mono 0.1g, poly 0.3g); PROTEIN 2g; CARB 50g; FIBER 5g; CHOL 0mg; IRON 1mg; SODIUM 26mg; CALC 21mg

Watermelon with Tangy Granita

1	cup water	¼	teaspoon crushed red pepper
¾	cup sugar	1	tablespoon grated lime rind
½	cup fresh lime juice	1	cucumber, peeled and seeded
⅓	cup packed mint leaves	8	cups (¾-inch) cubed watermelon
⅓	cup packed cilantro leaves	½	teaspoon kosher salt
¼	teaspoon kosher salt		

1. Combine 1 cup water and sugar in a microwave-safe dish. Microwave at HIGH 2 minutes; cool completely. Place syrup, juice, and next 6 ingredients (through cucumber) in a blender; blend until smooth. Pour mixture into an 11 x 7–inch glass or ceramic baking dish; cover and freeze 3 hours or until firm, stirring with a fork every 45 minutes. Remove mixture from freezer; scrape entire mixture with a fork until fluffy.
2. Place watermelon cubes in a large bowl. Sprinkle with salt; toss to combine. Let stand 10 minutes. Spoon about 1½ cups watermelon mixture into each of 6 bowls; top each serving with about ½ cup granita.

YIELD | SERVES 6

CALORIES 170; FAT 0.4g (sat 0g, mono 0.1g, poly 0.1g); PROTEIN 2g; CARB 43g; FIBER 1g; CHOL 0mg; IRON 0mg; SODIUM 244mg; CALC 25mg

Cantaloupe Granita

4	cups cubed peeled cantaloupe	2	tablespoons fresh lime juice
⅓	cup agave nectar	⅛	teaspoon salt

1. Place cantaloupe in a food processor or blender; process until smooth. Strain through a fine sieve over a bowl; discard solids. Stir in nectar, juice, and salt. Pour mixture into an 8-inch square glass or ceramic baking dish. Freeze at least 8 hours. Remove mixture from freezer; scrape entire mixture with a fork until fluffy.

YIELD | SERVES 4 (SERVING SIZE: ABOUT 1 CUP)

CALORIES 136; FAT 0.3g (sat 0.1g, mono 0g, poly 0.1g); PROTEIN 1g; CARB 35g; FIBER 1g; CHOL 0mg; IRON 0mg; SODIUM 100mg; CALC 15mg

PART 3

LIVING THE
GLUTEN-FREE
LIFESTYLE

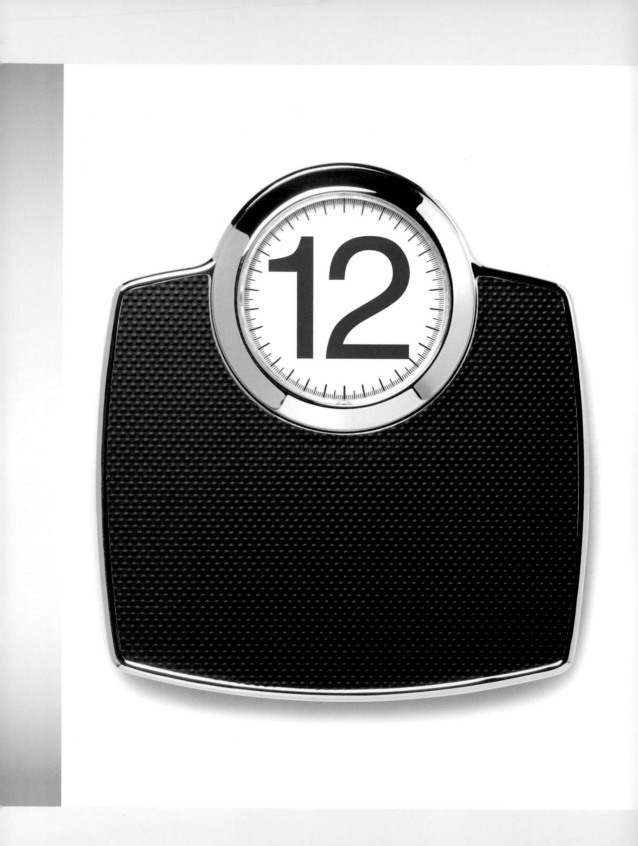

F YOU REALLY WANT TO BENEFIT from your gluten-free diet, exercise is a necessary step. As you shift your diet to this approach, your body will crave and respond to a routine that helps you get—and stay—fit. You'll be happy to learn that you won't have to trudge on a treadmill for hours or start scheduling marathons. In fact, if you're a regular exerciser you'll discover in these pages that you can probably exercise for less time *and* get better results.

Pairing your pure-energy eating plan with this fitness approach will do wonders for your body and your weight loss. The first step is to start building more activity into your typical day. For example, if you work in an office, try out a standing desk. Or, if that's not possible, look for opportunities to stand and move whenever possible. This could mean taking all your calls while standing or answering interoffice messages in person. Instead of tapping out an email or instant message, get up and walk over to your correspondent. You'll not only get more activity, but your officemates will probably appreciate the face-to-face contact.

As for actual exercise, make it your goal to find active ways to play so that your workouts never feel like an obligation. The problem with our modern-day exercise is that it's usually one more chore out of many, and we happily put it off when something—anything—better presents itself. For that reason, you'll want to find activities that you love so much that you can't bear *not* doing them.

The reason playing games—or just playing—works so well is that it usually involves quick bursts and brief rests. Think about most of the physical games we play: Tennis, racquetball, basketball, soccer—they all require quick explosive efforts broken up by brief rests. The great thing about this approach to exercise is that you can include tag and wrestling with the kids or a pet. The ideal exercise involves brief intense bursts, like running after a ball or pursuing someone, that are broken up with pauses in the action that allow you to catch your breath, such as when you're between points or rallies or while you're taking a break on the grass.

Why is this start-stop approach important? Researchers have found that breaking up your activity like this leads to more weight loss and improved fitness. Exercise scientists refer to this type of exercise as HIIT: high-intensity interval training. In study after study, researchers have found it far outperforms standard, steady-paced cardio. Another plus is that exercising this way is more fun.

In a 2011 study published in the *Journal of Obesity*, researchers reviewed all the research available on HIIT, or interval-based exercise, and found that it trumped steady-paced exercise in all the measures studied. Interval training increased fitness and fat loss more than regular exercise, and it accomplished these results in about half the time. (A typical interval-based workout runs 20 to 30 minutes, while steady-paced sessions usually run 40 to 60 minutes.) Even better for dieters, in one study, researchers found interval training led to at least three times the weight loss of steady-paced aerobics. Interval training also seems to target abdominal fat—your belly—which envelops organs and can lead to chronic disease.

There are more benefits to interval training. According to the American College of Sports Medicine, you can elevate your metabolism for up to 24 hours post-exercise by doing intervals. By injecting brief periods of intense effort into your exercise (either by playing fast-paced games or adding in some jogging and sprinting into your regular walks, runs, swims, or cycling), you can kick your metabolism up a notch during your workout—and it takes hours for it to slow down again. That equals ongoing calorie burn long after you've showered and toweled off.

Adding Intervals to Your Workout

Obviously, the best way to build in interval training is to pick up a sport that naturally requires brief bursts of intense effort. But you can't play tennis or basketball all the time. You may not even enjoy competitive sports.

Don't worry. You can still make intervals part of your workout by mixing them into your usual pursuit. If you're a walker and you typically exercise for 30 minutes, every five minutes try adding a burst of jogging or fast walking for 30 seconds. As you become more fit, you can increase the interval length to a minute and decrease the walking segments to four minutes. For the biggest metabolism boost, you'll want to make sure that the interval portion leaves you breathing hard. (By the way, if you haven't been exercising regularly, check with your doctor before you start an interval program.)

You can set a goal of working toward a more challenging interval sequence, at least according to science. Referred to as "10-20-30"—or more accurately, "30-20-10"—the concept is that after a proper warmup, you do 30 seconds of whatever your activity—walking, jogging, swimming, etc.—at a light, easy-to-maintain pace. Then do 20 seconds of normal-level intensity, and end the minute with 10 seconds of all-out effort before going back to 30 seconds of light effort. The advantage of this approach is that after five to 10 minutes, you'll get a very thorough and demanding workout. You can go longer, of course, but just 10 minutes of this leads to improved stamina and lower blood pressure and cholesterol, according to the Danish researchers at the University of Copenhagen who developed this approach.

Beef Up Your Exercise

The other important aspect of any exercise program is building strength. All activity prescriptions from fitness experts include strength training. Again, there's news here that will help you shorten the length of time you spend lifting while providing you with better results. This program will shape and tone your body while helping you shed more pounds—and keep them off.

Instead of doing three sets of light lifts and spending hours and days in the gym, think about doing briefer, more intense weight lifting. You don't even need equipment; you could use the resistance provided by your own body weight to create a complete full-body regimen. Push-ups, pull-ups, crunches, lunges, squats, and calf raises, and you're done.

However, many people find that going to a gym can help them stay committed to a program. Check out Bodypump or cardio-strength classes to simulate the kind of strength regimen you're looking for, or explore more old-school techniques like using kettlebells or CrossFit.

Strength training definitely helps you shed pounds faster while making your body look better. In 2010, Australian researchers reported that when overweight dieters added strength training three times a week, they lost much more weight than people who only dieted. After four months, the strength-training group had dropped an average of 30 pounds—10 pounds more than dieters. What's more, the lifters shaved 5.5 inches off their waistlines, compared to just 3.5 inches in the diet-only group. The exercises included just eight moves: shoulder, chest, tricep, and leg presses; seated rows; knee extensions; lat pull-downs; and sit-ups. You can approximate most of these lifts (or variations of them) at home with a pair of dumbbells.

Pulling off a workout with these kinds of benefits may mean lifting heavier weights than most people typically do (or want to). How much weight is enough? In the program below, you'll do two sets of each move. You should choose a weight heavy enough so that your muscles are spent after the second set.

Complete two sets of eight to 12 repetitions with a one-minute rest between sets. Schedule workouts at least twice a week, but make sure you have a day off between sessions to give your muscles a chance to recover.

1. Chest press
2. Dumbbell lunge
3. Shoulder press
4. Crunches

5. Calf raises
6. Dumbbell squat
7. Biceps curl
8. Triceps kickback

Chest press

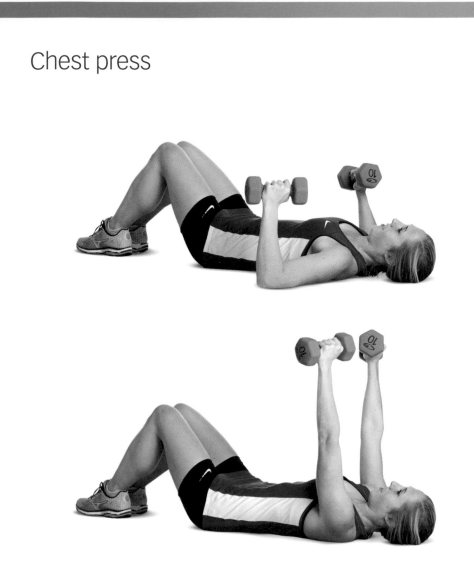

1. Lie on the floor faceup with your feet firmly on the ground, your back relaxed. Grasp a pair of dumbbells and with arms bent hold the dumbbells above your chest with your palms facing forward and your thumbs wrapped around each weight.

2. Exhale and slowly press the dumbbells straight up so they are over your shoulders. Wrists should remain in a neutral position (do not bend them throughout the exercise). Be careful not to arch your back. Inhale as you slowly lower the dumbbells back to starting position.

Dumbbell lunge

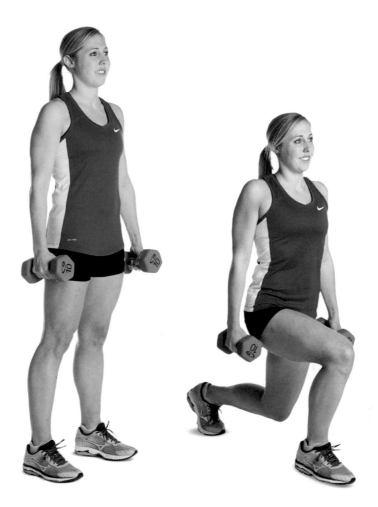

1. Stand with your feet hip-width apart, toes facing forward. Grasp a light dumbbell in each hand. Brace your torso by contracting your abdominal muscles. Slowly step forward with the right leg, placing your foot firmly on the ground. Keep your torso upright.

2. Inhale and bend your knees to lower your body toward the floor. Lunge only as far as you feel comfortable or until your right thigh is parallel to the floor. Now, exhale and firmly push off with your right (front) leg and return to your starting position. Repeat with the left leg.

Note: This exercise can also be done without weights.

Shoulder press

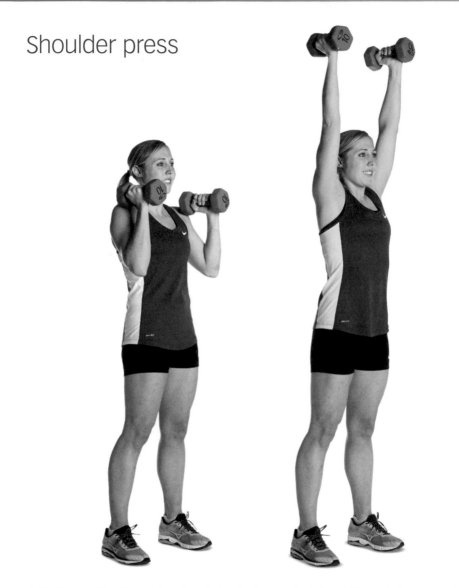

1. Hold a dumbbell in each hand, and stand with your feet hip-width apart. Brace your torso by contracting your abdominal muscles. Exhale and slowly lift the dumbbells until they are level with your shoulders. Palms should be facing in and thumbs should be wrapped around the handles. Wrists should remain in a neutral position (do not bend them throughout the exercise). Pull your shoulder blades down and back.

2. Exhale and press the dumbbells overhead until your elbows are straight, taking care not to arch your back. Inhale and slowly lower the dumbbells to shoulder height.

Crunches

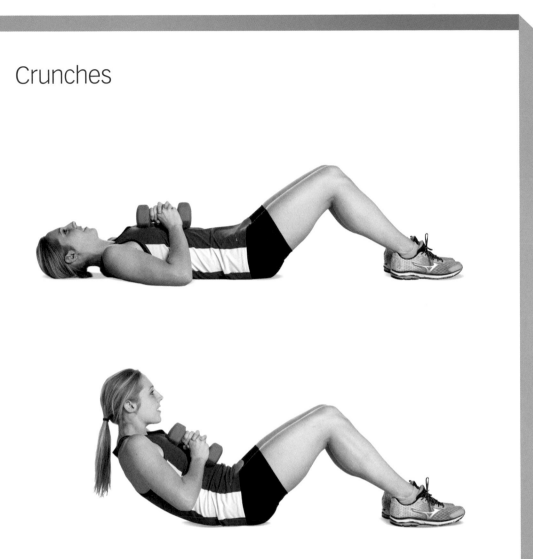

1. Lie faceup on the floor with your knees bent, feet flat on the floor, and heels a comfortable distance away from your rear. Grasp a dumbbell vertically against your chest with both hands.

2. Engage your abdominal muscles and exhale as you slowly raise your head and shoulders off the floor and draw your rib cage toward your pelvis. Continue until your mid back is lifted off the floor. Pause at the top of the motion; then slowly lower your head and shoulders back to the mat as you inhale. Repeat for 60 seconds.

Note: This exercise can also be done without weights.

Calf raises

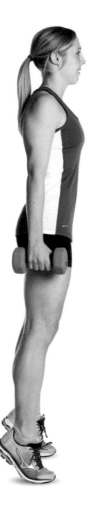

1. Stand holding a dumbbell in each hand. Spread your feet so they are hip-width apart. Keep your back straight and tighten your abs.

2. Exhale and slowly rise onto the balls of your feet, keeping your knees straight but not locked. At the top, pause and squeeze your calves. Inhale and lower yourself to the ground. Repeat step 2.

Note: This exercise can also be done without weights.

Dumbbell squat

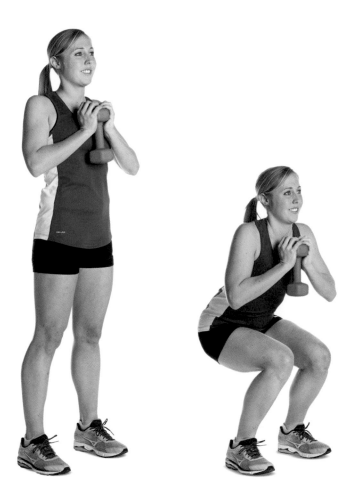

1. Grasp a dumbbell vertically in front of your chest with both hands, and point elbows to the floor. Spread feet until they are hip-width apart.

2. Inhale and squat by slowly pushing back your hips and bending your knees. Squat only as low as you feel comfortable or until your thighs are parallel to the floor. Pause; then exhale and slowly return to starting position.

Note: This exercise can also be done without weights.

Biceps curl

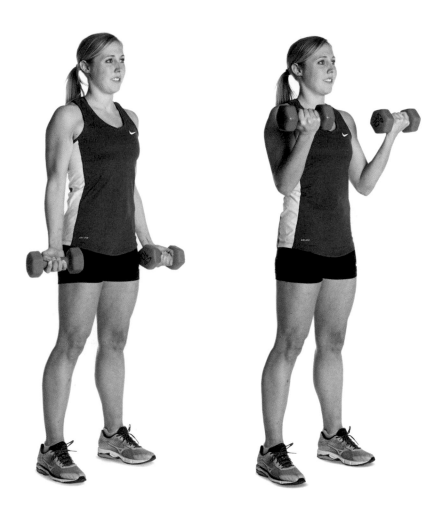

1. Stand with your feet hip-width apart and grasp a pair of dumbbells with palms facing forward and your thumbs wrapped around each weight. Keep your back straight, your abdominals tight, and your shoulders down and back.

2. Bending at your elbows, exhale and pull the dumbbells directly up until they are level with the top of your chest. Pause at the top of the movement. Inhale and slowly lower the dumbbells to the starting position.

Triceps kickback

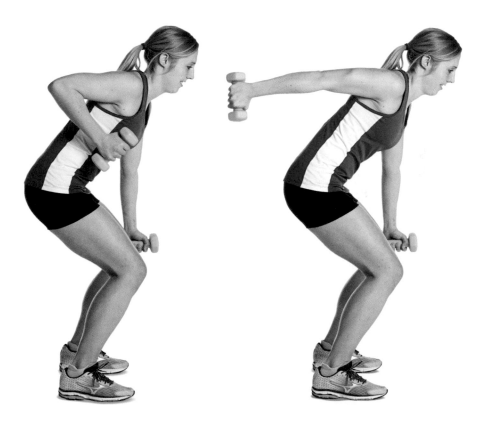

1. Grasp a pair of dumbbells with palms facing toward each other, thumbs wrapped around each weight. Spread your feet so they are hip-width apart and lean slightly forward, allowing dumbbells to hang.

2. Exhale and bend your right elbow and draw the dumbbell up to your side, making your upper arm parallel with the floor. Extend the dumbbell back to bring your forearm in line with your upper arm. Inhale and reverse the movement slowly by bending your elbow. Do 12 to 15 reps with each arm.

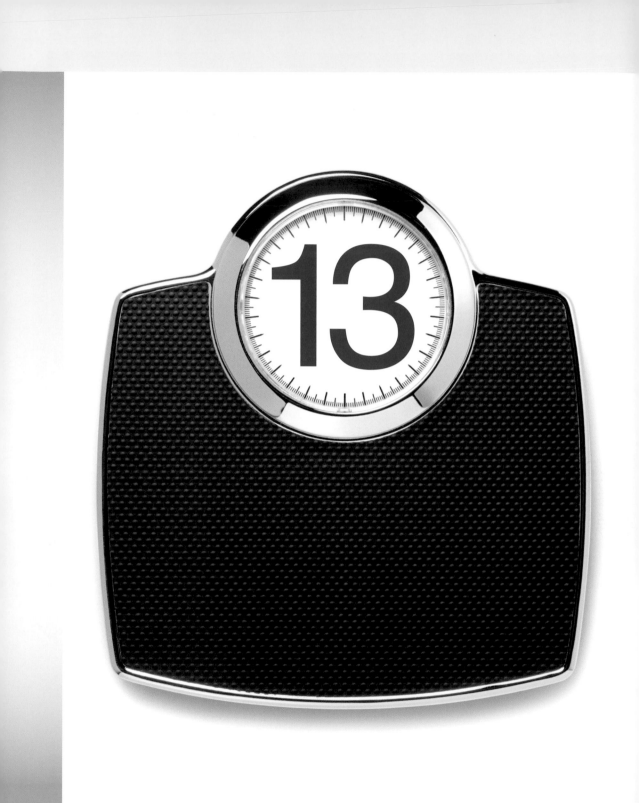

MAINTAIN YOUR GAINS
THE GLUTEN-FREE WAY

ONE OF THE MOST **COMMON DOWNFALLS** of successful dieters is thinking that maintaining weight loss will draw on the same skills it took to lose the weight in the first place. Unfortunately, that's just not true. According to health statistics from the CDC, only 20 percent of the people who go on a diet manage to maintain their weight loss for more than a year.

The trouble is that the skills we rely on to lose weight aren't all that useful when it comes to maintaining our weight loss. A 2011 national survey from researchers at universities around the United States—Penn State, Drexel, Ohio State, Stanford, and Texas—has found several distinct strategies to losing weight, and they're different from the ones we need to keep the pounds off.

Published in the *American Journal of Preventive Medicine*, the study suggests it's not simply a lack of willpower or self-control. Christopher Sciamanna, M.D., the study's lead author, queried 1,165 people about the behaviors they relied on to lose weight and, among those who were successful losers (they had kept off at least 10 percent of their weight for a year or more), how they had maintained that loss. Sciamanna and his colleagues found that out of 36 specific practices used for short-term and long-term weight loss, 14 were specific to either the dieting phase or the maintenance phase, but not both. Yet these were the most valuable strategies, since they were most likely to predict success in either losing weight or keeping it off.

Nearly every study shows that weight loss peaks and regain starts at six months, points out Sciamanna, a professor of medicine and public health at Penn State College of Medicine. He's hopeful that the study findings can alter this pattern. While many of the key practices sound familiar, Sciamanna's research is the first to distinguish the role each plays in weight loss versus weight maintenance. Several of the strategies Sciamanna looked at worked for both the active weight-loss phase and maintenance. These are the behaviors you'll want to learn early and retain for the rest of your life:

- Eating plenty of lean sources of protein, like fish, lean beef, and poultry
- Eating plenty of fruits and vegetables
- Limiting carbohydrates, especially junky ones such as chips and donuts
- Keeping careful control of portions
- Following a regular exercise routine
- Writing out—and sticking to—your grocery list
- Paying attention to nutrition labels and avoiding processed foods
- Reminding and rewarding yourself for reaching and sustaining a healthy weight
- Weighing yourself regularly

Sciamanna's findings on weight-loss strategies can serve as something of a road map to long-term success. But it's important to realize that you have to continue to pursue behaviors that will help you stay trim. Sciamanna points out that obesity is a chronic illness like hypertension; no one is surprised when a hypertensive patient stops taking her medication and her blood pressure rises, so it should be no surprise that when you stop using weight-control practices the weight will come back all the same, he says. We'll explore these valuable techniques and how they relate to your plan.

Keep Eating Gluten Free?

Once the weight comes off, you may be wondering whether you can or should continue to follow a gluten-free plan. After all, you're omitting big food groups—do you need to abandon them for life?

You may not need to be quite as strict about your gluten-free diet down the road—it all depends on how well the diet is working for you and how much you miss some of the foods you've given up. The decision is entirely up to you. If you're really craving bread, try adding a serving or two a week to see how your body responds. Try it for breakfast on a Monday and pay close attention to what your body does: If you find that you feel bloated later that day, you might want to continue avoiding gluten.

If you decide to have a sandwich with whole-wheat bread or sourdough, pay attention to how your stomach and digestive tract react over the next few hours. No problems? Good news—you can indulge in a sub every once in a while. However, if you feel bloated and your energy evaporates, you may want to stick with your gluten-free alternatives to satisfy your sandwich cravings.

And if at any time your weight starts creeping up, you'll want to eliminate the sources of gluten you've added back. The good news is that most people can manage a modified gluten-free eating approach while preserving their weight loss.

Keep Moving

If you're serious about avoiding weight regain, you'll need to stay active. One of the more robust research findings from the field of weight-loss maintenance has been the important role of regular exercise in keeping you slim. A study from the National Weight Control Registry found that people who were able to lose 30 pounds and keep it off for more than a year relied on a combination of diet and exercise; dieters who rely on one or the other aren't nearly as successful.

Lucky for you, you've already found the types of moves that keep you happy and engaged in staying fit; now you just have to be sure to make them a regular part of your life. That will mean staying injury free. One thing that will help is maintaining your strength, so continue to follow the strength-training regimen in Chapter 12. But you may also want to add a flexibility component to your exercise regimen. Regular stretching can keep your ligaments, tendons, and muscles pliable. A simple yoga routine can do wonders for your body, and it will help you release stress, which also plays a role in weight gain.

If you've never done yoga, check out a beginners class in your town or try a DVD at home. You'll soon come to love the way regular stretching feels. It can feel like lubricating your joints—you'll move easier, your performance during exercise will improve, and you'll experience less soreness when you're finished. Just remember to start slowly and go easy on your body. If you've never tried this type of stretching before, you may discover that your joints are nowhere near as flexible as those of the other participants in class or the instructor on your DVD. Don't worry about that, and definitely don't try to mimic or keep up with these people. Listen to your body, and only bend as far as feels comfortable. With time, you'll become much more flexible (although some people never attain the kind of flexibility on display in most yoga classes).

By the way, if you're looking for motivation to keep eating more protein than you once did, a study from a couple of years ago shows that a diet high in protein suits your exercise efforts. Remember the old canard about carb-loading before you exert yourself? Turns out it isn't nearly as effective as protein-loading. Researchers at the University of Stirling in Scotland asked cyclists to follow two identical three-week training sessions. The first week was normal effort, the second week was intensified training, and the third week was a recovery period. During the first session, the cyclists consumed a high-protein diet (about 1.5 grams of protein per pound of bodyweight); during the second session they ate normal meals with normal protein content—about half that of the high-protein diet—and made up the difference with carbohydrates.

On the high-protein regimen, the athletes not only performed better, but they also recovered faster after the intense training sessions. The athletes also reported feeling stronger when they got more protein. In other words, to get the most out of your exercise—and to bring your best effort—eat protein.

Simple Portion Control

Take a look in your cupboard. Those Frisbee-sized dinner plates and helmet-sized cereal bowls aren't doing you or your family any favors. The sad truth is that we eat what's put in front of us, regardless of how much there may be. Brian Wansink, a behavioral psychologist at Cornell University, has tested this in numerous ways. (One of his most devious experiments was a soup bowl that could continuously be filled surreptitiously from the bottom. Sitting around a table, volunteers engaged in conversation would continue to eat as long as there was soup in the bowl, no matter how full they felt.) Wansink has found that reducing your plate size by just 2 inches in diameter can reduce the amount of calories you take in by as much as 25 percent. Choose smaller cereal bowls and you'll get the same effect. Accounting for just breakfast and dinner, you could eliminate 350 calories a day. You could lose a pound every 10 days by doing this alone.

Shop Smart

As you have no doubt come to realize, a grocery list is invaluable when you're following a gluten-free plan. To maintain your loss, you'll want to keep your kitchen well stocked with gluten-free foods. For that reason, you'll always want to go through your kitchen before shopping to replenish any of the staples that are running low.

However, you may also want to start experimenting with new gluten-free foods. When you do, it will be helpful to make sure you understand the various labels on food packaging. Here's a quick guide:

"Low Sodium," "Reduced Sodium"

"Low sodium" means the product has to deliver fewer than 140 milligrams per serving. But "reduced sodium" just means that you're getting 25 percent less than the original item. If a food is extremely high in sodium already, like most canned soups, hitting the reduced-sodium bar is relatively easy. And if a manufacturer is reducing the salt content, it might be jacking up the sugar or fat content to boost flavor.

"Contains Real Fruit"

Sadly, these labels rarely say how much real fruit the food contains. You'll find this kind of label on fruit candy, sugary drinks that seem like orange juice, and other junky foods that are looking for the healthy stamp of approval to help harried moms feel better about buying the snack for children. Do yourself and your family a favor and check the number of sugar grams per serving. Compare brands and choose the item that has the lowest amount of sugar. (Be sure to check the serving size as well. If the package or bottle is something your child would finish in one sitting, but the nutrition label says it contains more than one serving, put it back on the shelf. The manufacturer has split up the servings because this food has too much sugar, fat, or calories in it.) The best way to get your fruit is in its original form, or by juicing it yourself at home. Skip the packaged stuff at the store.

"All Natural"

Food manufacturers trying to jump on the organic bandwagon coined this term. Unfortunately, it's meaningless. Unlike the term "organic," the government has very loose definitions for the term "all natural," and it can be slapped on any number of products that contain not-so-natural ingredients, according to the Center for Science in the Public Interest. The group found that products with the "all natural" labeling included teas sweetened with high-fructose corn syrup, chickens injected with high-sodium broth, and juices with artificial dyes. Don't be fooled by this wording.

Reward Yourself

Let's face it. You're putting in a lot of hard work losing weight and adapting to a new way of eating. So when you shed some pounds, indulge yourself. Shop for some new clothes, or give yourself a night out at a restaurant that can handle your gluten-free needs. Maybe you need a tennis racket or new exercise shoes. Set a weight goal, and when you hit it, give yourself a treat.

A Quick Restart

A great trick to keep your weight in check is keeping a food diary, which will be discussed more in depth in the next chapter. Any time you begin regaining weight, one of the first things you can try is restarting your food diary. This will help you track your gluten-free versus gluten intake. You may discover that you've let several forbidden foods creep back into your meals.

You may also discover that some new stress is pushing you to eat more, such as a new job, money pressures, or troubles with your kids. If emotions are driving you to overdo it, the quickest way to recognize and correct the problem is to use that food diary.

If things really get out of hand, try going through the four-week plan again. You'll quickly shed any pounds you may have regained, and you'll get a refresher course in gluten-free eating.

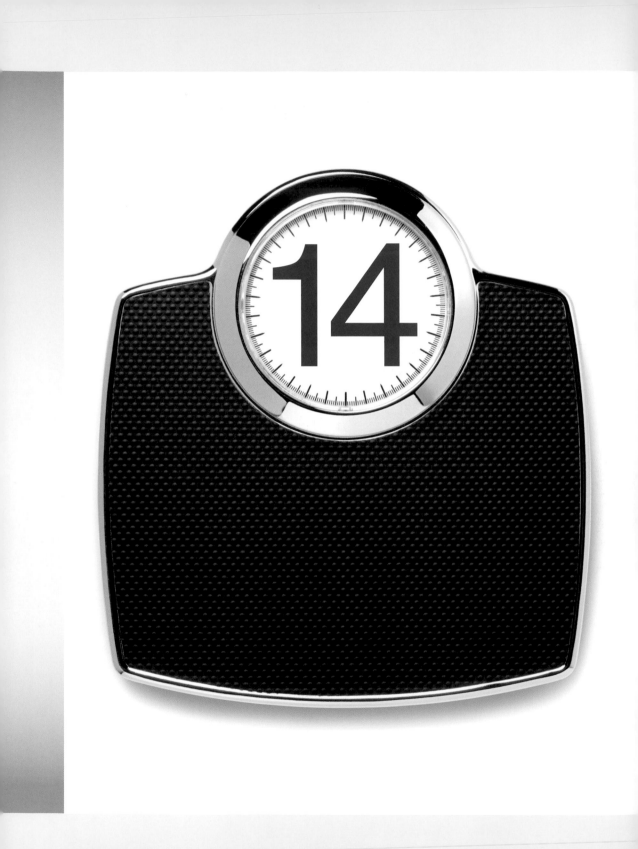

WHEN YOU'RE LOSING weight or trying to maintain your weight loss, you can't beat a little journaling to help you get a handle on the way you eat. A food diary is a powerful ally in your war on weight.

Studies demonstrate that the food diary is a very consistent and reliable contributor to weight loss. As it turns out, the simple act of writing down what you ate will make you more conscious of your intake and help you avoid overeating. Do it for the first four weeks of the diet and you'll naturally become more conscious of your eating habits and choices.

Keeping a food diary can serve another purpose: divining how much of your eating may be driven by your emotions. That's why there are entries for your mood on the diary pages that follow. Tracking *when* and *why* you eat may be as important to weight loss as tracking what you put on your plate. By cooking more and keeping gluten-free food and snacks around the house you can be sure that, when you eat, you'll choose food that will satisfy you and support your efforts to lose. But you'll also need to rein in urges to eat that are driven by stress, anger, loneliness, and other emotions.

For the next several weeks, keep the following diary pages with you. When you go to grab something to eat, record your emotional state. Are you bored? Are you upset about something that just happened? Are you mulling over a slight from earlier in the day? Then go ahead and eat, but halfway through, stop and make note of how you're feeling after you've had some food.

After a week, flip back through the journal and zero in on the times you saw a distinct improvement in your mood once you began eating. You've identified your emotional eating triggers, and now you can look for ways to replace the urge to eat with a healthier outlet for your feelings. A brisk walk, a phone call to a friend or loved one, taking time for some deep breathing, or simply chewing gum could make a big dent in your calorie intake.

Perhaps one of the most interesting aspects of keeping a food journal while on a gluten-free plan is that you'll find that you're thinking about eating much less than you once did. After a week or two, flip back through your journal and note how your eating habits have changed!

DAY OF WEEK	TIME OF DAY	MEAL

What are you eating?	
How hungry are you?	
Where are you?	
Describe your mood.	

DAY OF WEEK	TIME OF DAY	MEAL

What are you eating?	
How hungry are you?	
Where are you?	
Describe your mood.	

DAY OF WEEK	TIME OF DAY	MEAL

What are you eating?	
How hungry are you?	
Where are you?	
Describe your mood.	

DAY OF WEEK	TIME OF DAY	MEAL

What are you eating?	
How hungry are you?	
Where are you?	
Describe your mood.	

DAY OF WEEK	TIME OF DAY	MEAL

What are you eating?	
How hungry are you?	
Where are you?	
Describe your mood.	

DAY OF WEEK	TIME OF DAY	MEAL

What are you eating?	
How hungry are you?	
Where are you?	
Describe your mood.	

DAY OF WEEK	TIME OF DAY	MEAL

What are you eating?	
How hungry are you?	
Where are you?	
Describe your mood.	

DAY OF WEEK	TIME OF DAY	MEAL

What are you eating?	
How hungry are you?	
Where are you?	
Describe your mood.	

DAY OF WEEK	TIME OF DAY	MEAL

What are you eating?	
How hungry are you?	
Where are you?	
Describe your mood.	

DAY OF WEEK	TIME OF DAY	MEAL

What are you eating?	
How hungry are you?	
Where are you?	
Describe your mood.	

DAY OF WEEK	TIME OF DAY	MEAL

What are you eating?	
How hungry are you?	
Where are you?	
Describe your mood.	

DAY OF WEEK	TIME OF DAY	MEAL

What are you eating?	
How hungry are you?	
Where are you?	
Describe your mood.	

DAY OF WEEK	TIME OF DAY	MEAL

What are you eating?	
How hungry are you?	
Where are you?	
Describe your mood.	

DAY OF WEEK	TIME OF DAY	MEAL

What are you eating?	
How hungry are you?	
Where are you?	
Describe your mood.	

DAY OF WEEK	TIME OF DAY	MEAL

What are you eating?	
How hungry are you?	
Where are you?	
Describe your mood.	

DAY OF WEEK	TIME OF DAY	MEAL

What are you eating?	
How hungry are you?	
Where are you?	
Describe your mood.	

DAY OF WEEK	TIME OF DAY	MEAL

What are you eating?	
How hungry are you?	
Where are you?	
Describe your mood.	

DAY OF WEEK	TIME OF DAY	MEAL

What are you eating?	
How hungry are you?	
Where are you?	
Describe your mood.	

DAY OF WEEK	TIME OF DAY	MEAL

What are you eating?	
How hungry are you?	
Where are you?	
Describe your mood.	

DAY OF WEEK	TIME OF DAY	MEAL

What are you eating?	
How hungry are you?	
Where are you?	
Describe your mood.	

DAY OF WEEK	TIME OF DAY	MEAL
What are you eating?		
How hungry are you?		
Where are you?		
Describe your mood.		

DAY OF WEEK	TIME OF DAY	MEAL
What are you eating?		
How hungry are you?		
Where are you?		
Describe your mood.		

DAY OF WEEK	TIME OF DAY	MEAL
What are you eating?		
How hungry are you?		
Where are you?		
Describe your mood.		

DAY OF WEEK	TIME OF DAY	MEAL
What are you eating?		
How hungry are you?		
Where are you?		
Describe your mood.		

DAY OF WEEK	TIME OF DAY	MEAL

What are you eating?	
How hungry are you?	
Where are you?	
Describe your mood.	

DAY OF WEEK	TIME OF DAY	MEAL

What are you eating?	
How hungry are you?	
Where are you?	
Describe your mood.	

DAY OF WEEK	TIME OF DAY	MEAL

What are you eating?	
How hungry are you?	
Where are you?	
Describe your mood.	

DAY OF WEEK	TIME OF DAY	MEAL

What are you eating?	
How hungry are you?	
Where are you?	
Describe your mood.	

Nutritional Information

HOW TO USE IT AND WHY

The following is a helpful guide to put the nutritional analysis numbers into perspective. Remember, one size doesn't fit all, so take your lifestyle, age, and circumstances into consideration when determining your nutrition needs.

IN OUR NUTRITIONAL ANALYSIS, WE USE THESE ABBREVIATIONS

sat saturated fat	**poly** polyunsaturated fat	**CHOL** cholesterol	**g** gram
mono monounsaturated fat	**CARB** carbohydrates	**CALC** calcium	**mg** milligram

DAILY NUTRITION GUIDE

	Women ages 25 to 50	Women over 50	Men ages 24 to 50	Men over 50
Calories	2,000	2,000 or less	2,700	2,500
Protein	50g	50g or less	63g	60g
Fat	65g or less	65g or less	88g or less	83g or less
Saturated Fat	20g or less	20g or less	27g or less	25g or less
Carbohydrates	304g	304g	410g	375g
Fiber	25g to 35g	25g to 35g	25g to 35g	25g to 35g
Cholesterol	300mg or less	300mg or less	300mg or less	300mg or less
Iron	18mg	8mg	8mg	8mg
Sodium	2,300mg or less	1,500mg or less	2,300mg or less	1,500mg or less
Calcium	1,000mg	1,200mg	1,000mg	1,000mg

The nutritional values used in our calculations either come from The Food Processor, Version 10.4 (ESHA Research), or are provided by food manufacturers.

Metric Equivalents

The information in the following charts is provided to help cooks outside the United States successfully use the recipes in this book. All equivalents are approximate.

COOKING/OVEN TEMPERATURE

Farenheit	225°F	250°F	275°F	300°F	325°F	350°F	375°F	400°F	425°F	450°F	475°F	500°F
Celsius	110°C	120°C	135°C	150°C	160°C	180°C	190°C	205°C	220°C	230°C	245°C	260°C

LENGTH
(To convert inches to centimeters, multiply the number of inches by 2.5.)

1 in =	2.5 cm
6 in = ½ ft =	15 cm
12 in = 1 ft =	30 cm
36 in = 3 ft = 1 yd =	90 cm
40 in =	100 cm = 1 m

LIQUID INGREDIENTS BY VOLUME

1 tsp =			1 ml
3 tsp = 1 Tbsp =	½ fl oz =	15 ml
2 Tbsp = ⅛ cup =	1 fl oz =	30 ml
16 Tbsp = 1 cup =	8 fl oz =	240 ml
1 pt = 2 cups =	16 fl oz =	480 ml
1 qt = 4 cups =	32 fl oz =	960 ml
	33 fl oz =	1000 ml = 1 l

DRY INGREDIENTS BY WEIGHT
(To convert ounces to grams, multiply the number of ounces by 30.)

1 oz =	¹⁄₁₆ lb =	30 g
4 oz =	¼ lb =	120 g
8 oz =	½ lb =	240 g
12 oz =	¾ lb =	360 g
16 oz =	1 lb =	480 g

References

CHAPTER 1: GLUTEN FREE AND YOUR HEALTH

Murray JA. *Mayo Clinic Going Gluten Free: Essential Guide to Managing Celiac Disease and Related Conditions.* Birmingham: Oxmoor House. 2014.

Davis JL. The Risks of Belly Fat. WebMD. www.webmd.com

Atkinson SA, Josse AR, Phillips SM, Tarnopolsky MA. Increased consumption of dairy foods and protein during diet- and exercise- induced weight loss promotes fat mass and lean mass gain in overweight and obese premenopausal women. *Journal of Nutrition*. 2011; 141: 1626-1634.

Aller EE, Larsen TM, Claus H, Lindroos AK, Kafatos A, Pheiffer A, Martinez JA, Handjieva-Darlenska T, Kunesova M, Stender S, Saris WH, Astrup A, van Baak MA. Weight loss in overweight subjects on ad libitum diets with high or low protein content and glycemic index: the Diogenes trial 12-month results. *International Journal of Obesity*. 2014; 38: 1511-1517.

Dietary Guidelines for Americans, 2010. www.dietaryguidelines.gov

Voegtlin, WL. *The Stone Age Diet*. New York: Vantage Press, Inc. 1975.

CHAPTER 2: WHY GOING GLUTEN FREE IS GOOD FOR YOU

Cordain L. *The Paleo Diet: Lose Weight and Get Healthy by Eating Foods You Were Designed to Eat.* New Jersey: John Wiley & Sons, Inc. 2002, 2011.

Layman DK, Evans EM, Erickson D, Seyler J, Weber J, Bagshaw D, Griel A, Psota T, Kris-Etherton. A moderate-protein diet produces sustained weight loss and long-term changes in body composition and blood lipids in obese adults. *Journal of Nutrition*. 2009; 139: 514-521

The Paleo Diet. www.thepaleodiet.com

Mark's Daily Apple. www.marksdailyapple.com

CHAPTER 12: EXERCISING FOR GLUTEN-FREE HEALTH

Boutcher SH. High-intensity exercise and fat loss. *Journal of Obesity*. 2011; 2011: 868305

Trapp EG, Chisholm DJ, Freud J, Boutcher SH. The effects of high-intensity intermittent exercise training on fat loss and fasting insulin levels of young women. *International Journal of Obesity*. 2008; 32: 684-691

For All-Day Metabolism Boost, Try Interval Training. American College of Sports Medicine. www.acsm.org

Wycherley TP, Noakes M, Clifton PM, Cleanthous X, Keogh JB, Brinkworth GD. High-Protein Diet with Resistance Exercise Training Improves Weight Loss and Body Composition in Overweight and Obese Patients with Type 2 Diabetes. *Diabetes Care*. 2010; 33: 969-976

When to See a Doctor. American College of Sports Medicine. www.acsm.org

Physical Activity and Health. Centers for Disease Control and Prevention. www.cdc.gov

CHAPTER 13: MAINTAIN YOUR GAINS THE GLUTEN-FREE WAY

Sciamanna CN, Kiernan M, Rolls BJ, Boan J, Stuckey H, Kephart D, Miller CK Practices Associated with Weight Loss Versus Weight-Loss Maintenance. *Preventative Medicine*. 2011; 41: 159-166

Wansink B. Why Visual Cues of Portion Size May Influence Intake. Cornell University Food and Brand Lab. www.foodpsychology.cornell.edu

Index

A

Alcoholic drinks, 44
Amaranth
    Vanilla Amaranth with
        Peach Compote, 76
Amylopectin A, 25
Arteries, inflammation of, 19
Artificial sweeteners, 40–41
Autism, 18

B

Baking sheets, 47
Barley, 24, 44
Beans
    Black Bean Soup, 105
    Bourbon Baked Beans, 156
    Five-Bean Chili, 135
    Portobello and Black Bean
        Quesadillas, 103
    Simmered Pinto Beans with
        Chipotle Sour Cream, 157
    Spicy Bean and Quinoa Salad
        with "Mole" Vinaigrette, 90
    Tomato-Basil Pasta
        with Asiago, 141
Beef
    Banh Mi–Style Roast Beef
        Sandwiches, 97
    Cast-Iron Burgers, 118
    Slow-Cooker Brisket, 117
    Spicy Steak Lettuce Wraps, 95
    Stuffed Poblanos, 137
Beer, 44
Belly fat, 13–14, 191
Blenders, 48–49
Bread, unhealthful ingredients in, 25
Breakfasts, 69–84
Buckwheat
    Savory Buckwheat with Tomato,
        Cheddar, and Bacon, 77

C

Carbohydrates, 13–14, 15, 16
Casein, 17–18
Celiac disease, 12, 17, 57, 64
Chicken
    Blueberry Chicken Salad, 94
    Braised Chicken with
        Honey-Lemon Leeks, 131
    Chicken-Olive Quesadillas, 102
    Chicken Verde Enchiladas, 130
    Chicken with Turnips and
        Pomegranate Sauce, 126
    Citrus-Herb Chicken, 124
    Dijon-Herb Chicken Thighs, 134
    Greek-Style Chicken Breasts, 129
    Grilled Chicken Thighs with
        Cilantro-Mint Chutney, 132
    Roasted Carrot, Chicken,
        and Grape Quinoa Bowl, 93
    Shredded Chicken Tacos with
        Tomatoes and Grilled Corn,
        127
    Spicy Chicken Sandwiches, 99
    Spicy-Sweet Chicken Lettuce
        Cups, 100
Chickpeas
    Warm Brown Rice and Chickpea
        Salad with Cherries and Goat
        Cheese, 92
Cholesterol, 19
Cilantro-Mint Chutney, 132
Cookies and bars
    Almond-Date Bars, 175
    Amaretti, 181
    Lemon Sugar Cookies, 179
    Maple-Pecan Bars, 176
    Peanut Butter–Chocolate Chip
        Cookies, 180
Cooking utensils, 45–49
Cross-contamination, 34, 40, 47, 59
Cutting boards, 48

D

Dairy-free products, 18
Dessert options, gluten-free, 56
Desserts
    Blackberry-Almond Cobbler, 169
    Blueberry Cheesecake
        Ice Cream, 183
    Butterscotch Pudding, 173
    Cantaloupe Granita, 185
    Cherry-Grapefruit-Basil
        Sorbet, 182
    Chocolate–Peanut Butter
        Pudding, 173
    Cocoa Cupcakes, 168
    Grilled Peaches with
        Honey Cream, 170
    Jasmine Chai Rice
        Pudding, 174
    Lemon Verbena–Buttermilk
        Sherbet, 181
    Meyer Lemon Panna Cotta, 172
    Pineapple Upside-Down
        Cake, 167
    Quick Berry Frozen Yogurt, 182
    Raspberries with Peach-Basil
        Sorbet, 184
    Watermelon with Tangy
        Granita, 185
Diet soda, 40–41
Dinners, 108–143

E

Eating on the run, 58
Eating out, 57
Egg poachers, 46
Eggs
    Mexican Chorizo Hash, 73
    Mushroom Frittata, 70
    Peppery Potato Omelet, 69
    Zucchini and Red Pepper
        Frittata, 71

Exercise

Exercise
    flexibility component, 206
    increase in daily activity, 190
    interval training, 190–191
    strength training, 192–193
    weight lifting program, 193–201

F

Fast food, 23, 24
Fats, 19
Fish
    Cedar Plank Salmon with Tomato
        Salsa, 110
    Saffron Rice with Tilapia and
        Shrimp, 111
    Salmon Salad on Arugula, 89
    Salsa Flounder, 108
    Sautéed Tilapia Tacos with Grilled
        Peppers and Onion, 114
    Tilapia Veracruz, 113
    Tuna-Pecan Salad Sandwiches, 94
Flexibility, 206
Flours, gluten-free, 32–36
Food diary, 212–219
Food plans, 52–55
Food processors, 48
Foods
    to avoid, 40
    gluten-free, 31
    may be gluten-free, 36–37
Fruit
    Cantaloupe Granita, 185
    Cherry-Grapefruit-Basil
        Sorbet, 182
    Mozza Fruit Skewers, 150
    Peach Compote, 76
    Raspberries with Peach-Basil
        Sorbet, 184
    Watermelon with Tangy
        Granita, 185

G

Gluten, defined, 12
Gluten-free diet
    advantages of, 12–13
    gluten-free foods, 31
    health benefits of, 17–18, 24–26
    maintaining, 205–206, 209
    "maybe" foods, 36–37
    nutrients in, 26
    shopping list for, 64–65
    websites, about gluten-free
        lifestyle, 64
    weight loss and, 12–14
Gluten-free products, 23, 30
Gluten sensitivity, 12, 17, 22
Grains, gluten-free, 31
Graters and zesters, 46

H

High-protein diet, weight loss and,
    13–14, 16, 26–27
High-protein diet plans, 19

HIIT (high-intensity interval training), 190–191
Hormone overload, 25
Hunger, 16–17, 25

I

Inflammation, 19, 25
Insulin, rise in, 13
Interval training, 190–191

K

Knives, 46

L

Labels, decoding, 38, 208–209
Lactose intolerance, 18
Leptin, 25
Lunches, 89–105

M

Measuring cups, 45
Measuring spoons, 46
Metabolism, elevating, 191
Mixers, electric, 48
Mushrooms
    Portobello and Black Bean
        Quesadillas, 103

O

Oat flour, making, 83
Oats
    Blueberry-Almond Oatmeal
        Pancakes, 81
    Cinnamon, Apple, and Oat
        Scones, 84
    Mixed Berry Muffins, 83
    Oatmeal Pancake Mix, 80
    Oatmeal Pancakes, 80
    Oatmeal Waffle Mix, 80
    Pecan-Oatmeal Waffles, 82
    Pumpkinseed-Almond
        Granola, 75
    Sunflower Granola, 75
Obesity, 13–14, 205

P

Pasta
    Pasta Carbonara Florentine, 143
    Pasta with Roasted Red Pepper
        and Cream Sauce, 142
    Three-Cheese Baked Penne, 140
    Tomato-Basil Pasta with
        Asiago, 141
    Vegetarian Lasagna, 139
Polenta
    Goat Cheese and Basil
        Polenta, 161
Pork
    Pork Tenderloin and Cannellini
        Beans, 121
    Pork Tenderloin with Roasted
        Cherries and Shallots, 123
    Pork Wraps with Fresh Tomatillo
        Salsa, 98

Roasted Pork Tenderloin
    Tacos, 119
Portion control, 207
Potassium bromate, 25
Potatoes
    Cheesy Hash Brown
        Casserole, 74
    Lemon-Caper Parmesan Potato
        Salad Bites, 159
    Pan-Seared Mojo Potatoes, 160
    Peppery Potato Omelet, 69
    Rustic Garlic Mashed
        Potatoes, 161
Processed food, eliminating, 22–23
Produce, benefits of, 23
Protein, 13–14, 16, 26–27

Q

Quinoa
    Breakfast Quinoa, 79
    Quinoa with Strawberries and
        Buttermilk, 77
    Roasted Carrot, Chicken, and
        Grape Quinoa Bowl, 93
    Spicy Bean and Quinoa Salad
        with "Mole" Vinaigrette, 90

R

Research
    on artificial sweeteners, 40–41
    on digestive tract, 24
    on high-protein diet, 13–14,
        26–27, 207
    on hunger, 25
    on interval training, 192
    on low-fat diets, 19
    on portion control, 207
    on strength training, 192–193
    on weight loss and maintenance
        strategies, 204–205
Rice
    about, 37
    Asian Rice with Shrimp and
        Snow Peas, 116
    Garlic-Parmesan Rice, 162
    Warm Brown Rice and Chickpea
        Salad with Cherries and Goat
        Cheese, 92
    Wild Rice with Squash, 162
    Yogurt Rice with Cumin and
        Chile, 163
Rye, 24, 44

S

Scales, kitchen, 45
Scallops
    Seared Scallops with Snap Peas
        and Pancetta, 115
Shopping list, 64–65
Shrimp
    Asian Rice with Shrimp and
        Snow Peas, 116
    Saffron Rice with Tilapia and
        Shrimp, 111

Skillets, cast-iron, 47
Slow cookers, 49
Snack options, gluten-free, 56
Snacks
    Cheddar-Bacon-Chive Dip, 148
    Edamame Crunch, 150
    Green Goodness Dip, 149
    Lemon-Parmesan Popcorn, 151
    Mozza Fruit Skewers, 150
    Roasted Garlic and Chive
        Dip, 146
Soda, 40–41
Spices, gluten-free, 44
Spiralizer, 46
Stockpots, 48
Storage containers, 49
Strength training, 192–193

T

Thermometers, digital, 46
Thyroid, effect of bread on, 25
Travel, gluten-free diet and, 59
Turkey
    Sausage Pizza, 138

V

Vegetables
    Beet–Blood Orange Salad, 155
    Bourbon Baked Beans, 156
    Broccoli-Cheese Soup, 104
    Browned Butter and Lemon
        Brussels Sprouts, 153
    Cabbage Slaw with Mango
        Vinaigrette, 153
    Caprese Zucchini, 155
    Pan-Charred Asparagus, 152
    Sautéed Green Beans with
        Spice-Glazed Pecans, 154
    Vegetarian Lasagna, 139
    Wild Rice with Squash, 162

W

Websites, gluten-free lifestyle, 64
Weight lifting program, 193–201
Weight loss
    benefits of, 19
    gluten-free diet and, 12–13
    high-protein diet and, 13–14, 16
    interval training and, 190–191
    maintaining, 204–205
Wheat
    allergies, 17–18
    difficulty in digesting, 24
    leptin, 25

Y

Yoga, 206

©2015 by Time Inc. Books
1271 Avenue of the Americas, New York,
    NY 10020

ISBN-13: 978-0-8487-4483-0
ISBN-10: 0-8487-4483-7
Library of Congress Control Number: 2015933187
Printed in the United States of America
First Printing 2015

Be sure to check with your health-care provider
before making any changes in your diet.

Oxmoor House
Editorial Director: Anja Schmidt
Creative Director: Felicity Keane
Art Director: Christopher Rhoads
Executive Photography Director: Iain Bagwell
Executive Food Director: Grace Parisi
Photo Editor: Kellie Lindsey
Managing Editor: Elizabeth Tyler Austin
Assistant Managing Editor: Jeanne de Lathouder

The 10 Pounds Off Gluten-Free Diet
Senior Editor: Betty Wong
Editor: Rachel Quinlivan West, R.D.
Editorial Assistant: April Smitherman
Assistant Test Kitchen Manager:
    Alyson Moreland Haynes
Recipe Developers and Testers: Julia Levy,
    Stefanie Maloney, Callie Nash, Karen Rankin
Food Stylists: Nathan Carrabba,
    Victoria E. Cox, Margaret Monroe Dickey,
    Catherine Crowell Steele
Senior Photographer: Hélène Dujardin

Senior Photo Stylists: Kay E. Clarke,
    Mindi Shapiro Levine
Production Manager: Theresa Beste-Farley
Assistant Production Director: Sue Chodakiewicz

Contributors
Writer: John Hastings
Assistant Project Editor: Melissa Brown
Designer: Ben Margherita
Junior Designer: AnnaMaria Jacob
Copy Editors: Dolores Hydock,
    *Marra*thon Production Services
Proofreader: Kate Johnson
Indexer: *Marra*thon Production Services
Nutrition Reviewer: Barbara Linhardt, R.D.
Fitness Reviewer: Michele Stanten
Fellows: Laura Arnold, Kylie Dazzo, Nicole Fisher,
    Loren Lorenzo, Anna Ramia, Caroline Smith,
    Amanda Widis

Time Inc. Books
Publisher: Margot Schupf
Vice President, Finance: Vandana Patel
Executive Director, Marketing Services:
    Carol Pittard
Executive Director, Business Development:
    Suzanne Albert
Executive Director, Marketing: Susan Hettleman
Assistant General Counsel: Simone Procas
Assistant Project Manager: Allyson Angle

Photo Credits
Courtesy of: 15 Carmen Kelly, before and
after; 39 Dorothy Herbst, before and after **Getty
Images:** 6, 10, 20, 28, 42, 50, 62, 66, 86, 106,
144, 164, 188, 202, 210 DNY59, scale; 34 Alasdair
Thomson, buckwheat; 37 Kadir Barcin, rice

Back cover
Left: Sautéed Tilapia Tacos with Grilled Peppers
    and Onion, page 114
Right: Shredded Chicken Tacos with Tomatoes
    and Grilled Corn, page 127